MANAGED CARE: INTEGRATING THE DELIVERY AND FINANCING OF HEALTH CARE

PART A

The Health Insurance Association of America
Washington, DC 20004-1109

ISBN 1-879143-26-7

TABLE OF CONTENTS

FOREWORD v

PREFACE vii

ACKNOWLEDGMENTS ix

Chapter 1
INTRODUCTION TO MANAGED CARE 1

Chapter 2
THE DEVELOPMENT OF MANAGED CARE 13

Chapter 3
ORGANIZATION OF MANAGED CARE ARRANGEMENTS 33

Chapter 4
COST CONTROL TECHNIQUES 55

Chapter 5
INDIVIDUALS, EMPLOYERS, AND MANAGED CARE 75

Chapter 6
GOVERNMENT INVOLVEMENT IN MANAGED CARE 91

Chapter 7
CONTROLLING FOR QUALITY 117

Chapter 8
DATA FOR QUALITY, COST, AND UTILIZATION CONTROL 139

Appendix A
HEALTH MAINTENANCE ORGANIZATION ACT OF 1973 157

Appendix B
HEALTH MAINTENANCE ORGANIZATION MODEL ACT 181

Appendix C
PREFERRED PROVIDER ARRANGEMENTS MODEL ACT 217

NOTES 221

GLOSSARY 227

INDEX 241

FOREWORD

The HIAA Insurance Education Program aims to be the leader in providing the highest quality educational material and service to the health insurance industry and other related health care fields.

To accomplish this mission, the Program seeks to fulfill the following goals:

1. Provide a tool for use by member company personnel to enhance quality and efficiency of services to the public;

2. Provide a career development vehicle for employees and other health care industry personnel; and

3. Further general understanding of the role and contribution of the health insurance industry to the financing, administration, and delivery of health care services.

The Insurance Education Program provides the following services:

1. A comprehensive course of study in Group Life and Health Insurance, Individual Insurance, Long-Term Care Insurance, and Managed Care;

2. Certification by examination of educational achievement for all courses;

3. Programs to recognize accomplishment in the industry and academic communities through course evaluation and certification, which enables participants to obtain academic or continuing education credits; and

4. Development of educational, instructional, training, and informational materials related to the health insurance and health care industries.

PREFACE

Over the past 40 years, the health and disability insurance industry has undergone many profound changes. As these changes have occurred, the HIAA Insurance Education Program has sought to incorporate them in its curriculum in order to achieve its mission of maintaining high-quality educational material and service.

A significant recent change affecting the health insurance industry is the integration of the administration and financing of health benefits with the delivery of health care services—managed care. The importance of managed care has warranted the development of new HIAA Education Program curriculum materials, and this text with its accompanying self-study manual is the first, Part A, of a two-text curriculum in Managed Care.

Successful completion of the Managed Care curriculum, in addition to courses from the Group Life and Health, Individual Health, and Long-Term Care curricula, will lead to the HIAA designation of Managed Healthcare Professional (MHP).

Many of the concepts contained in the Managed Care curriculum are constantly in flux. Characteristics evolve over time, and insurers and managed care organizations find themselves at different stages along a continuum of managed care programs. In addition, the insurance industry operates in an ever-changing regulatory climate. These realities are important to keep in mind during the study of HIAA's entire curricula.

The contents of this book are educational, not a statement of policy. The views expressed or suggested in this and all other HIAA textbooks are those of the contributing authors or editors. They are not necessarily the opinions of HIAA or of its member companies.

ACKNOWLEDGMENTS

Allison A. Alkire
Sanus Corp. Health Systems

Howard L. Bailit
Aetna Life and Casualty Insurance
Company

Ruth E. Baldwin
CNA Insurance Companies

Tamarra J. Burnicle
General American Life Insurance
Company

Jonathon M. Fuchs
Consultant

Mike Kohl
The Principal Financial Group

Gregory J. Koppe
General American Life Insurance
Company

Donald W. Kress
Healthsource Provident
Administrators, Inc.

Ted W. LaBedz
Humana Insurance Company

Mark Langenfeld
State Farm Mutual Automobile
Insurance Company

Terry Lowe
State Farm Mutual Automobile
Insurance Company

Nicoletta B. Morin
Massachusetts Mutual Life Insurance
Company

Gail Nachbaur
New York Life Insurance Company

Gail B. Neldon
New York Life Insurance Company

Martin Rosenbaum
The Great-West Life and Annuity
Insurance Company

Juliana L. Torma
New York Life Insurance Company

Chapter 1

INTRODUCTION TO MANAGED CARE

1 Introduction
1 Factors That Affect the Need for Developing Managed Care
2 Areas of Needed Change
8 Managed Care

9 Differences Between Traditional Indemnity Insurance and Managed Care
10 Summary
10 Key Terms

■ Introduction

Today's health care system is under intense scrutiny. America's employers, consumers, and policymakers are all seeking ways to curb continuing cost inflation and to expand access to care. Unless health care costs are better controlled, providing access to medical services for the more than 35 million Americans currently without health care coverage will be difficult. At the same time that cost and access are major concerns, many people also are grappling with difficult questions about medical decisions and quality of care provided. While there is disagreement about methods, most Americans agree that some reform or change in the health care system is necessary.

While the debate about health care reform continues, the free enterprise system in the United States has fostered development of new forms of health care delivery and financing that attempt to address many of these issues. This private enterprise development can be generally characterized as managed care. It is this evolving system of health care financing and delivery that is the subject of this course.

■ Factors That Affect the Need for Developing Managed Care

The United States has traditionally relied, in large part, on a private health care financing system, based on charging a premium and paying provider bills on a fee-for-service basis, that provides payment for defined benefits or covered loss. While this system has met with success in the past, there are acknowledged problems with its current operation. Medical services have become very expensive, and those who need protection are sometimes left uncovered. Generally, these problems are the consequence of:

- inappropriate or nonexistent incentives for providers and consumers to utilize the health care system efficiently;
- lack of coordination and integration in the management of chronic conditions or serious diseases or trauma;
- unrealistic public expectations of the health care system, coupled with lack of individual responsibility for maintaining a healthy lifestyle;
- proliferation of new, expensive technologies with unproven benefits;
- a shift to chronic, long-term care services necessitated by an increasing aging population and other demographic changes; and
- cost shifting from Medicare and Medicaid to privately insured patients to compensate for revenue lost, either because of lower fees paid by government or uncompensated care from those unable to pay.

Other contributing factors include:

- an excess of health care resources in certain geographic areas (called excess capacity);
- the practice of defensive medicine, where excessive and unnecessary services are delivered because of the fear of malpractice suits;
- fraud and waste;
- regulatory barriers to cost containment; and
- insufficient data to determine the best and most cost-effective course of treatment.

One way to attack these problems is to identify and correct the system's faults, while retaining the positive aspects of the system. This suggests that several aspects of the health care system will have to undergo change.

■ Areas of Needed Change

There is no simple solution to the problem of rising costs and their effect on the financing and delivery of health care services. Effective solutions require changes in fundamental attitudes, behaviors, and expectations on the part of consumers, providers, payers, and government. Changes also will need to occur in such areas as assessing and using technological advances and in recognizing a shift in demographics that places new demands on the health service system.

Reasons for Needing Consumer Changes

For the well insured, the decision to consume care is not a financial decision; cost is no object. The result can be high levels of consumption with tolerance of costly, and sometimes unnecessary and/or inefficient, medical service.

Americans have come to view access to health care as a right, a viewpoint insulated from the direct costs of care. They have tended to go one step further to assume that health care is a benefit that should not be conditioned by price or other socioeconomic constraints. As a consequence, Americans often believe that everyone should be able to consume care if there is any positive marginal benefit to be realized. They do not ask, as with other goods and services, whether the extra benefit justifies the cost.

The public's tendency to demand high levels of care is often exacerbated by poor response to prevention. Rather than take primary responsibility for maintaining their physical and biological systems, they often assume that the medical system will cure any health problems that may arise. Expectations are often unrealistic regarding the medical system's ability to repair damage that abuse, or simply the passage of time, has caused. Americans typically expect that no expense will be spared to remedy the problem. Again, the consequence is greater pressure to increase the level of health expenditures.

Finally, consumers are at a disadvantage as the complexities of modern medical diagnosis and treatment have forced them to turn over many important decisions to physicians. Even with incentives to be economical, they often lack the knowledge to make informed decisions. Because consumers can neither manage the medical maze nor understand what services are needed, they let physicians and other providers make health care decisions for them.

Reasons for Needing Provider Changes

Physicians play a key role in determining what medical resources are used. Once an individual decides to seek care, physicians either strongly influence, or directly make, most of the decisions that determine the cost of care. Unfortunately, most physicians have had neither the knowledge nor the incentive to be concerned about cost. In fact, the fee-for-service system of payment that dominates physician reimbursement rewards physicians for providing more, not less, care. As long as the amount physicians earn is directly determined by the number of services they provide or order for their patients, it will be difficult to keep health care costs from rising. The problem does not lie just with the small minority of physicians who are consciously trying to maximize reimbursement by manipulating the system in their favor. Noneconomic incentives—the desire to please patients and to convince them that they are receiving high-quality treatment, the pressure to reduce uncertainty, the threat of malpractice suits, the desire to use the newest technology—push even the most scrupulous physician in the direction of doing more than providing only necessary and effective care.

Even if the physician reimbursement system did not produce perverse incentives and waste, physicians might not always be able to provide care in the most cost-effective way. Often they must act without adequate knowledge. To choose the most cost-effective course of treatment for any medical problem, a physician must be able to identify that course of treatment. Unfortunately, until recently, information on state-of-the-art treatment rarely distinguished between cost-effective and costly forms of diagnosis and therapy. In other cases, the knowledge has not been disseminated widely or effectively enough to become standard practice. And in other instances, physicians may choose not to adopt more cost-effective procedures or treatments into their medical practice. Consequently, care is more costly than it should be.

Hospitals, too, are affected, particularly by the Medicare Prospective Payment System (PPS). (Chapter 2) Hospitals are concerned about the long-term effects of PPS, such as a decrease in inpatient volume, a shift to outpatient settings, and difficulties with maintaining or expanding their medical staff. In particular, hospitals want to protect their relationships with the specialists that admit patients. These specialists, in turn, are concerned about having a sufficient level of clinical work to support their hospital practice and protect their earnings. To retain specialists, hospitals are attempting to protect and broaden their physician referral base, which serves as a feeder system to the institution. Hospitals and specialists have been placed in the position of seeking alternatives to the traditional system of referral such as risk-sharing contracts.

Reasons for Needing Payer Changes

The present health care delivery system continues to be composed of many independent providers working without formal mechanisms for coordinating the delivery of care. Such an arrangement is neither efficient nor in the patient's best interest. It frequently leaves no single provider in charge of managing all aspects of the patient's care. The traditional fee-for-service reimbursement system has rewarded providers in proportion to the amount of service they provide. Such economic incentives encourage expensive patterns of medical practice. Without monitoring or constraints, such an arrangement is bound to produce high-cost care.

By simply paying the bills, as the traditional fee-for-service insurance system has done, consumers have been encouraged to use the system in an inefficient way, with little regard or understanding of costs. When all or most medical bills are paid directly by the insurer to the provider, the consumer has little incentive to examine cost-effectiveness or comparative quality of service.

Another problem with the traditional fee-for-service indemnity insurance system is high administrative costs. The traditional insurance system has created an environment that fosters diversity, choice, and flexibility. Such an environment inevitably means that there will be a loss of administrative economies of scale found in centrally financed or managed systems. The high cost of administration has affected the ability of small groups or employers to afford private health insurance for their employees. As a result, working people are left uninsured, which has undesirable social consequences.

Traditional insurance also has directed its payment system at the treatment of disease rather than at prevention or early intervention. Benefit plans rarely paid for physicals and other preventive care and, in fact, generally paid more generous benefits for expensive hospital or specialist care than for outpatient, primary care. The tendency for the system to emphasize care for illness over health maintenance has helped to increase both health costs and a reliance on more intensive methods of health care.

New Approaches to Technological Advances

Within the medical care system is an environment of constantly changing technology, which exacerbates the cost problem. Medical advances today generally do not have dramatic potential for curing or preventing a major category of disease. Instead, even though technologically sophisticated and extraordinarily complex, these advances tend to improve only marginally the ability to treat disease. Often they are diagnostic technologies that advance the ability to identify medical problems without adding greatly to the capacity to improve patients' health.[1] The new technologies also can use more resources than they replace. Some are clearly beneficial in improving patient welfare by reducing pain and risk; others contribute little to improved health status. The proliferation of new technologies reflects Americans' general tendency to place excessive reliance on technology and medical intervention to manage health problems. Evidence actually shows only a weak link between health status and levels of spending for medical services, and reveals that lifestyle and environmental conditions often have a greater impact on health status than use of the medical system.[2] The cost of continued demand for new technology has been substantial over the past decade.

Need for Government Changes

Many aspects of government activity affect the cost and utilization of health care services. Some of the more prominent are examined below.

Legislative/Regulatory Barriers

Government action sometimes contributes to, rather than helps, the cost problem. Regulations, particularly at the state level, sometimes prohibit insurers and others from implementing promising cost-containment efforts.[3] These cost-containment efforts may involve innovative arrangements with providers, financial incentives for consumers to choose efficient providers, or effective forms of utilization review.

Mandated Benefits

State regulations that mandate coverage for specific diseases, provider groups, or categories of medical services often add to insurance costs.[4] Rather than outline general requirements for basic health care benefits that can be managed, many states, through pressure from special interest groups, require that all health insurance benefit packages include specific services or specific categories of providers. Frequently, such services are of a questionable benefit and can be costly.

Litigation

The current legal environment has led to the practice of defensive medicine. The threat of suits appears to encourage physicians to provide more services than they would if they did not fear being sued for malpractice. In addition, the cost of litigating and settling those disputes that go to court adds to malpractice premium costs, which are ultimately translated into higher provider fees. States that do not seek to place limits on malpractice awards and awards for punitive damages contribute to the cost inflation of medical practice.

Data Deficiencies

Inadequate data are another cause of rising health care costs. Data deficiencies often limit:

- insurers' and payers' ability to monitor provider performance;
- understanding of how one medical market performs compared with others; and
- analysis of the cost-effectiveness of accepted, new, and emerging technologies and standards of practice.

Some data elements that are necessary to manage the delivery of care effectively are either not collected at all or are not captured consistently in provider or insurer databases. In addition, the data that are collected are often not in a standardized format, so that information from different sources cannot be combined and compared to provide an accurate picture of the system as a whole. The failure of the federal government to assume a leadership role in defining common data collection formats has contributed to a more costly and less efficient health care system. This failure has also led to inconsistency, as individual states take the lead in establishing state-specific data requirements that are not necessarily compatible with those of other states.

In addition to an inability to make use of common statistical input for planning and cost controls, insurers have found that a lack of standardized databases makes abuse and fraud in the health care system easier. Though many states have insurance fraud bureaus, it often can be a tedious and difficult process to identify instances of providers defrauding insurers for their own financial gain.

Government Cost Shifting

The enactment of Public Law 89-97 in 1965 ushered in a new era for the federal government and state governments to finance the nation's health care services. This federal statute created the Medicare and Medicaid programs. Medicare was designed to help pay for the health care services of people age 65 and over. Medicaid was established as a jointly financed federal-state program to provide health care benefits for the poor of all ages.

Because the cost of Medicare and Medicaid is far greater than predicted when the programs were developed, federal and state governments have developed various methods of limiting payment to health care providers, including tightening regulations for determining reimbursable costs. As a result, hospital and physician payments for Medicare and Medicaid are significantly lower than prevailing charges. Medicare and Medicaid patients by law are charged less than private-pay patients. To the extent that health care providers seek to make up this loss of income, cost shifting from the public programs to the privately insured will continue to be a health care cost inflation factor for those with private insurance.

Supply of Health Resources

The supply of certain health resources in the United States has expanded rapidly, but without the discipline usually provided by the laws of supply and demand. The result, according to observers,[5] is an excess supply of physicians, hospital beds, and expensive technologies, all of which have contributed to excessive costs. In spite of the large increase in physician supply, the distribution of physicians from one region of the country to another remains uneven. Although the supply of many specialties and subspecialties is far greater than needed, particularly in urban areas, the supply of primary care physicians remains inadequate to meet medical needs in many geographic areas.[6] Little action has been taken that match medical resources to need.

The Need to Respond to Changing Demographic Needs

The population of the United States is aging rapidly. During the 1980s, the number of Americans over 65 years of age increased by 22 percent to 12 percent of the total population. By the year 2025, it is estimated that over 18 percent of the population will be over age 65.[7] The age group growing most rapidly is senior citizens 85 years and older.[8] This group makes greater use of the health care system than other age groups. In addition, because of chronic or debilitating diseases related to the aging process, their health care often includes more high-cost services, rehabilitation, or care and medication use over a long period of time.

The development of technological advances has prolonged the lives of people who would have died from accident or illness in the past. These people often require extensive rehabilitation and continuing treatment for the remainder of their lives.

One other area of chronic care where utilization has increased during the past fifteen years is treatment for mental illness. The advent of new interventions, programs, and medications has fostered an increase in demand for mental health care.

These demographic increases in chronic care groups have placed greater demand on the health care system. This demand is followed by an increase in supply of services that, in turn, causes an increase in health care costs.

◼ Managed Care

The health care system has changed substantially over the last decade and continues to evolve. As mentioned previously, this evolving system has inherent problems, particularly in the area of cost inflation. These problems require strategies to combat them. Increased development of managed care delivery systems is one solution that attempts to address many of the problems and issues listed above.

What Is Managed Care?

Because it is an evolving concept, there is no single, universally accepted definition of managed care. This book defines managed care as systems that integrate the financing and delivery of appropriate health care services to enrollees by means of one or more of the following elements:

- arrangements with selected providers to furnish a comprehensive set of health care services to enrollees;
- explicit standards for the selection of health care providers;
- formal programs for ongoing quality improvement and utilization review;
- an emphasis on keeping enrollees healthy to reduce use of services; and
- financial incentives for enrollees to use providers and procedures associated with the plan.

Common Features of Managed Care

Most managed care systems include the following six features:

1. rigorous utilization review;
2. monitoring and analysis of the practice patterns of physicians;
3. use of primary care physicians and other caregivers to manage patients;
4. steering of patients to high-quality, efficient providers;
5. quality improvement programs; and
6. reimbursement systems that make physicians, hospitals, and other providers financially accountable for the cost and quality of medical services.

The underlying principle is that responsibility must be taken to manage and integrate the whole range of services the patient needs. The fundamental objective is to reduce costs by promoting appropriate and efficient use of health care services.

■ Differences Between Traditional Indemnity Insurance and Managed Care

There are several fundamental differences between the operation and objectives of traditional indemnity insurance and managed care. (Figure 1.1)

Managed care, which integrates payment for health care with its delivery, is market-driven. Today's health care purchaser is demanding more control over costs, better quality care, accountability from providers, and fiscally sound,

Differences Between Traditional Insurance and Managed Care

Traditional Insurance	Managed Care
Has no restrictions on choice of providers	Encourages or requires use of selected providers
Offers fee-for service reimbursement of providers	Pays negotiated rates paid to providers
Functions apart from the health care delivery system	Integrates the finance and delivery system
Assumes all financial risk	Shares risk with providers
Offers few financial incentives to control costs	Creates financial incentives for providers and enrollees to control costs
Takes no interest in measuring quality and appropriateness of services	Participates actively in methods to measure quality and monitor appropriateness of care
Has no real budget for cost of services, simply "pay as you go"	Establishes budget for cost of services, prepayment of a fixed premium in many cases

Figure 1.1

efficient administration. Managed care now challenges insurers, who were once solely in the business of financing health care, to assume new roles. They must create systems that deliver health care to consumers, initiate new relationships with providers, and administer complex new organizations.

■ Summary

Employers, consumers, and policymakers are all seeking ways to curb rising health care costs and expand access to health care. The traditional method of using private, fee-for-service indemnity insurance has not proven to be effective in managing the rising health care costs of a changing health care system. The development of managed care concepts of integrating financing with service delivery is one way of addressing the need for changing the health care system. Private insurers are responding to the challenge of rising costs and poor access by attempting to incorporate the basic principles of managed care into current practice.

■ Key Terms

Appropriateness of care	Defensive medicine	Fee-for-service
Chronic care	Enrollees	Fraud
Cost shifting	Excess capacity	Incentives

Indemnity insurance
Malpractice
Managed care
Mandated benefits
Medicaid
Medical practice
   patterns

Medicare
Medicare Prospective
   Payment System (PPS)
Prepayment
Prevailing charges
Preventive medicine

Providers
Reimbursement system
Standard practice
Utilization
Utilization review

Chapter 2

THE DEVELOPMENT OF MANAGED CARE

13 *Introduction*

14 *Forerunners*

15 *Health Benefits During and After World War II*

17 *The HMO Act*

19 *The 1980s and 1990s*

21 *Insurer Response to Managed Care*

23 *The Current Managed Care Marketplace*

31 *Summary*

31 *Key Terms*

■ Introduction

Managed care has its origins in the traditional indemnity (or fee-for-service) insurance concept of prepaying for medical care services. Though the concept of insurance (the transfer of all or part of risk of loss in return for payment of a premium) goes back to ancient times, the modern American concept of group indemnity insurance began in the 20th century. In 1911, Montgomery Ward and Company negotiated an insurance plan to provide weekly benefits for its employees who were unable to work because of sickness or injury. Before this, employers organized the actual delivery of health services to employees rather than provide insurance.

The first medical service bureau was formed in 1917 in Tacoma, Washington, by doctors eager to contract with timber and mining companies. The first multispecialty group practice, the Mayo Clinic, was established at the turn of the century in Rochester, Minnesota, by a family of physicians who understood the efficiencies of group practice.

Over the years, changes in the economy of the United States stimulated many initiatives for health care financing and delivery. Several corporate giants that had emerged out of 19th-century industrialization quickly perceived that providing medical benefits might help them attract and retain a good work force. By the 1920s, major insurance companies were contracting with corporations to include group hospital care in employee insurance packages. The Depression, which made medical care unaffordable for millions of Americans, stimulated labor unions to contract directly with prepaid group practices. It also encouraged the extension of the corporate movement into health care.

■ Forerunners

There were several forerunners to current health care organizational and financial arrangements.

Hospital Insurance

In 1929, the principle of group prepayment for hospital expenses (premiums paid in advance for coverage for specific services) originated at Baylor University Hospital in Dallas, Texas. Some 1,500 school teachers, members of a mutual benefit society, were covered for 21 days of semiprivate room and board and necessary hospital services. The Baylor Plan is considered the forerunner of what later became known as the Blue Cross Plans, a program for providing protection against the costs of hospital care in a limited geographic area. These early plans specifically covered hospital care; thus they came to be known as "hospitalization plans."

Prepaid Group Practice

Also in 1929, Donald E. Ross, a former railroad surgeon, and H. Clifford Loos, formerly of the Mayo Clinic, founded the first prepaid group practice. A prepaid group practice plan is one in which specified health services are rendered by participating physicians to an enrolled group of persons. Fixed, periodic payments were made in advance by or on behalf of each person or family. This concept was the forerunner of the health maintenance organization (HMO), described in Chapter 3.

Ross brought to the partnership his experience with prepayment for medical services, while Loos was practiced in the Mayo's system of reviewing patient records and physician performance. The same year that the Ross-Loos Clinic was founded, Baylor University contracted with the university hospital for Baylor's faculty members.

Preferred Provider Organizations and Individual Practice Associations

In 1934, Southern California Edison formed the first selective provider relationships, a forerunner of preferred provider organizations (PPOs), by contracting with independent providers of all kinds, including hospitals, to provide health care for a fixed payment. PPO plans are explained more fully in Chapter 3. In the same decade, a group of Oregon doctors organized themselves into a fore-runner of the individual practice association (IPA) in order to compete against prepaid group practices. The IPA is a managed care plan built around physician associations. (Chapter 3) Their Physicians' Association of Clackamas County borrowed some of the features of prepaid groups, but its physicians were solo practitioners.

Health Maintenance Organizations

In 1938, the industrialist Henry J. Kaiser asked surgeon Dr. Sidney Garfield to start a group practice for his Grand Coulee Dam workers. When, after the outbreak of World War II, Kaiser opened shipyards to supply the war effort, Garfield organized hospitals and clinics to provide prepaid comprehensive health services to shipyard workers. The plans opened their membership to the public after the war. They are now known as the Kaiser Permanente Medical Care Program, the largest group-model HMO in existence today. (The group-model HMO contracts with a group or groups of providers who agree to provide services to HMO participants in exchange for a fee.)

■ Health Benefits During and After World War II

Employee benefits proliferated during the war. Benefits were a means of attracting skilled workers, who were in short supply, and absorbing excess profits. (A profit cap on manufacturing and general industry was in force.) After the war, enabling legislation and favorable changes in tax law encouraged the spread of group health benefits, which labor unions sought enthusiastically. In 1948, the National Labor Relations Board (NLRB) ruled that health benefits were a proper subject for collective bargaining. For the next 20 years, employer-paid health benefits spread to nonunion and professional workers and were consolidated into a single type of policy, known today as group medical catastrophe coverage. Such policies provide insurance against such catastrophic situations as prolonged hospital confinement and expensive medical procedures.

Opposition to Managed Care

Prepaid group practice and staff-model plans (HMOs that employ their own physicians) would have spread even more rapidly had they not been opposed by much of the medical establishment. The American Medical Association (AMA) and state and local medical societies were not sympathetic to managed care because they had no financial interest in its success. Believing that the prepaid group practices represented a threat to traditional fee-for-service medicine, they embarked on campaigns to prevent the successful operation of these group practices. Medical societies threatened group practice physicians with expulsion from the society and used their coercive power to deprive them of hospital privileges. However, in a 1943 case involving the AMA and the Medical Society of the District of Columbia, the Supreme Court was unanimous in its opinion that the medical societies had violated the Sherman Antitrust Act in conspiring to monopolize the field of medical practice.

The AMA rescinded its opposition to prepaid groups in 1949, but unofficial opposition from some special interest groups has continued. However, the growing number of physicians participating in managed care programs has blunted the effect of opposition somewhat. In fact, certain medical societies began organized efforts to assure that all physicians were given the right to participate in managed care, even if the managed care program did not want or need their participation.

Early Prepaid Plan Techniques

The early prepaid groups and IPAs that had generated so much controversy were practicing first-generation managed care techniques:

- the use of primary care physicians as gatekeepers (a primary care case management approach that requires authorization for medical services delivered by specialists);

- quality control through physician peer review (evaluation of physician practice, based on a set of criteria, conducted by other physicians);

- pre-approval for nonemergency hospitalization;

- alternatives to inpatient care (such as outpatient care, outpatient or same-day surgery); and

- second surgical opinions (a prospective screening process, relying on consulting physician's or surgeon's evaluation of the need for surgery by another surgeon).

These techniques proved that these early groups could contain treatment costs and they became attractive to employers concerned by inflated medical costs. Cost escalation, which began in the 1950s, accelerated in succeeding decades. By the 1970s, it was higher than that of the overall Consumer Price Index.

■ The HMO Act

The delivery of health care in the United States was revolutionized when, under pressure from health care reformers, the Nixon Administration introduced the HMO Act in 1973. (Appendix A) Passage of the HMO Act legitimized HMOs and encouraged their development throughout the nation by authorizing funds for grants and loans to develop new HMOs, by overriding state mandates restricting the development of HMOs, and by mandating that federally qualified HMOs could require large employers to offer at least one HMO to their employees.

Also, the HMO Act of 1973 established a voluntary certification process for HMOs. In return for becoming federally qualified under the Act, HMOs could require employers to offer the health plan as part of the employer's health benefits program. Initially, federally qualified HMOs were eligible for grants and loans. Many early HMOs became federally qualified as voluntary compliance was considered a seal of approval.

By the end of 1981, when funding for loans stopped, grants totaling $145 million had been awarded under the Act's authority for HMO feasibility, planning, and development purposes. In addition, HMOs received direct loans totaling $185 million and loan guarantees totaling nearly $9 million. However, the ambitious goal of creating 1,700 HMOs enrolling 40 million members was never reached.[9] The HMO Act funding was relatively short-lived. Employers remained reluctant, however, and the "HMO boom" envisioned at the outset never quite materialized. More recently, in part because of greater public acceptance of HMOs and changes in the Act, fewer HMOs are seeking to become federally qualified.

In addition to voluntary federal qualifications, state statutes regulate HMOs. Virtually every state has enacted some form of licensure law that incorporates a process for certification. HMO regulations can be found under a state's health code, insurance code, or both. It should also be noted that, in the early evolution of HMOs, the National Association of Insurance Commissioners (NAIC), an organization of state insurance commissioners, took the initiative in developing a model HMO Act for states. (Appendix B)

Beyond the HMO Act

By the late 1970s, employers were increasingly alarmed by the rising costs of their employees' health benefits. General Motors, for example, was paying more than $1 billion each year in health insurance premiums, which added $400 to the price of each GM car. Many employers recognized the potential for managed care systems to reduce these costs. At the same time, medical schools

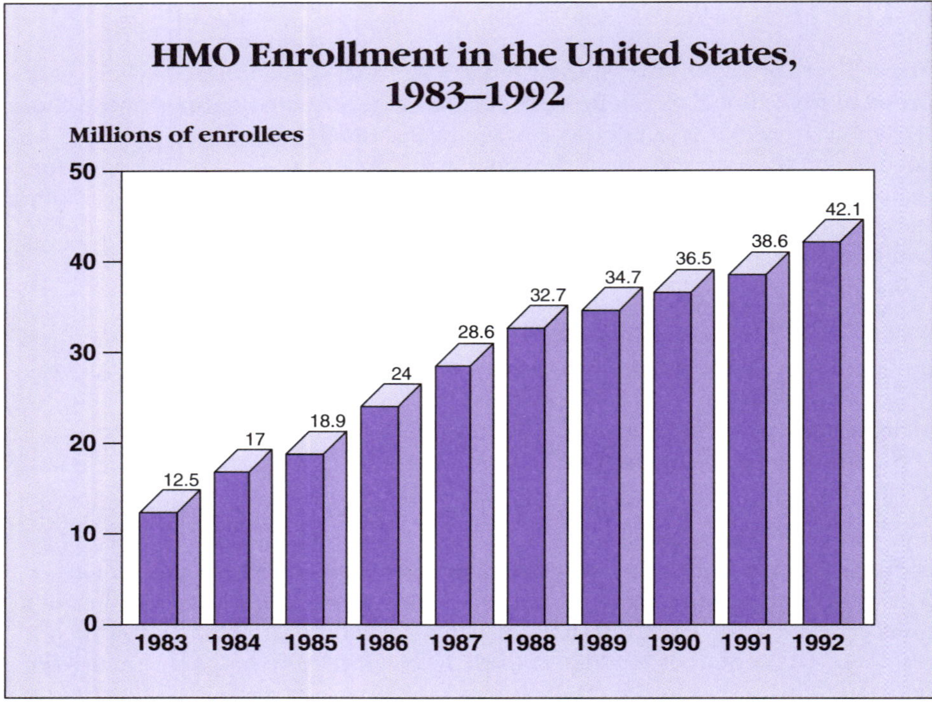

Figure 2.1

SOURCE: The InterStudy Competitive Edge, 1993.

were producing so many graduates that many highly qualified physicians were drawn into HMOs, dispelling myths that HMOs could not attract high-quality physicians.

Growth of Managed Care

From the mid-1970s to the 1990s, HMO enrollment grew at a rate of 25 to 30 percent each year. (Figure 2.1) IPA-model HMOs (Chapter 3) became increasingly popular for several reasons:

- They were less costly to develop than group-model HMOs because they operated out of the existing offices of independent physicians, reducing start-up costs.

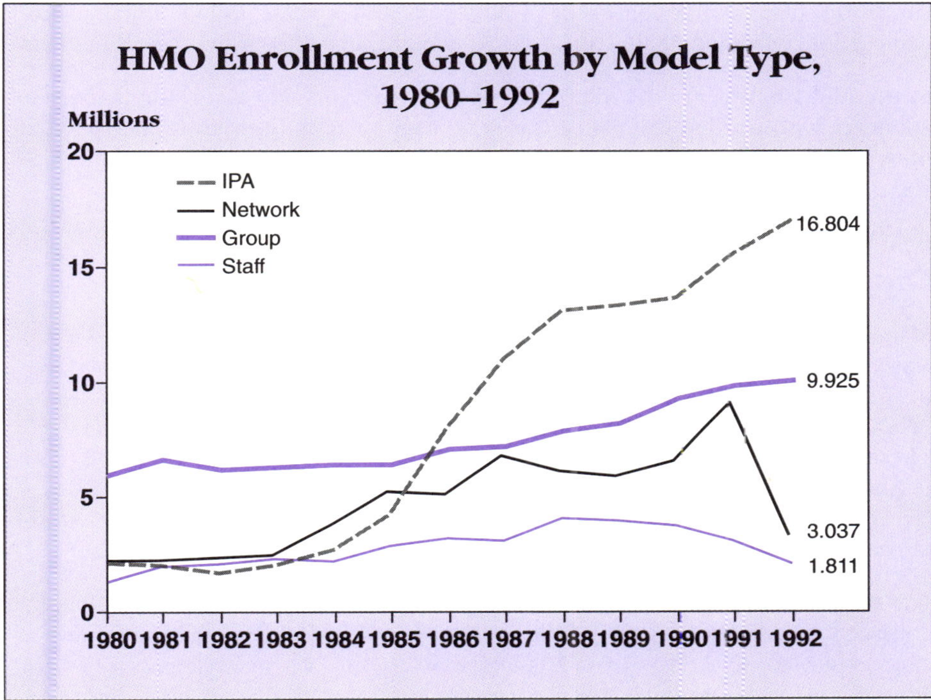

Figure 2.2

SOURCE: The InterStudy Competitive Edge, 1993.

- Physicians in private practice could affiliate with IPAs without having to become the salaried employees of groups; in fact, many physicians were affiliated with more than one HMO.

- Patients had access to community physicians in private offices in the surroundings with which they were most familiar. Some patients even found that their family doctor participated in the HMO in which they enrolled.

In the past decade, the IPA was the fastest-growing HMO model. (Figure 2.2)

■ The 1980s and 1990s

The growth in HMO enrollment in the 1970s resulted in a growing need to finance expansion. A number of not-for-profit independent plans and provider-sponsored plans converted to for-profit status, and several HMO companies became publicly traded chains, in order to acquire financing from capital markets.

In the mid-1980s came the first wave of HMO mergers and acquisitions, as plan sponsors who needed to finance the next stage of HMO growth found they had underestimated the necessary resources. HMO plans sponsored by providers sought buyers or partners for mergers and joint ventures.

Changing Perspectives

Managed care firms and independent third-party vendors began to incorporate successful managed care programs and techniques—such as utilization review, hospital bill audit, managed mental health and substance abuse programs, and managed pharmacy programs—into discrete products that they sold separately. These products and programs were, in essence, entirely new to the health care industry. As problem areas in health care delivery were identified, such specialization grew. Each time a new need was identified, a new industry (such as the utilization review industry) sprang up to address that need.

The first PPOs were formed in California, where the law permitted selective contracting with health care providers. PPOs are less tightly structured managed care plans and differ from IPA-type HMOs in two major respects: (1) They allow members to go outside the contracted network of providers with a reduction of benefits rather than a forfeiture of benefits; and (2) physicians and facilities offer fee-for-service discounts to the plan, but share no other risks. (Chapter 3) Because insurers believed that these features would be attractive to both providers and consumers, PPOs spread quickly outside California.

HMOs, eager to exploit the flexibility offered by PPOs, developed a hybrid product (the open-ended HMO) with which they could compete with PPOs. An open-ended HMO allows its members to use physicians outside the plan in exchange for additional personal financial liability in the form of a deductible, co-insurance, or copayment. Because most members use the network providers, these HMOs assume a limited additional financial risk. Group Health of Minneapolis offered open-ended HMO coverage as early as 1961, and it was the success of this type of plan in Minnesota that encouraged HMOs in other parts of the country to offer open-ended coverage. HMOs in some states were prevented by state law from taking on financial risk for out-of-plan care. They were forced to join with insurers to devise "wrap-around" coverage. Such experiments led to the development by carriers of point-of-service (POS) plans, which have gained considerable support from employers who view them as cost management programs that also have flexibility. A POS plan is one that offers a managed care arrangement but allows the insured to obtain services outside the managed care plan at the time service is sought, for higher out-of-pocket cost. (Chapter 3)

Membership in HMOs grew from 3 million in 1970 to 18.9 million in 1985.[10] By 1986, competition was producing premium price wars. Only HMOs that had maintained sufficient reserves, adequate premiums, and effective medical management escaped financial instability during this time period. A study conducted by the HMO Solvency Working Group of NAIC concluded that the probable reasons for HMO insolvencies in 1988 were:

- inadequate initial capital and surplus;
- absent or ineffective utilization controls;
- inadequate premium rates;
- inadequate permanent capital and surplus; and
- inadequate budgeting and estimation of expenses.

In other words, organizations that suffered insolvencies were weak in the areas of financing and in medical, actuarial, and executive-level management.

Because the HMO is both a health care delivery system and a financing system, it requires the infrastructure and expertise appropriate to both. Successful HMOs were the ones that could incorporate systems for marketing, medical management, provider relations, quality assurance, network management, data collection and analysis, rating, and actuarial, financial, and general administration.

■ Insurer Response to Managed Care

Many insurers entered the managed care market during the merger and growth period of the mid-1980s. They recognized the need to respond to the growing managed care phenomenon. Traditional health insurance companies made acquisitions and engaged in new development activities in order to remain competitive and retain market share in a changing health care market. The entrance into managed care was also inspired by the success of managed care programs in controlling health care costs. Employers, seeing profits eaten away by the cost of health benefits, pressured insurers to develop stronger, more effective cost control features.

Insurers' first entry into managed care was through experimentation with HMOs. Either they assumed financial liability for the plan or, less frequently, when employers were self-insured, undertook its claims processing and benefits administration. Because PPOs did not require the significant start-up investment that HMOs demand, early on insurers became more heavily committed to this model, which more closely resembled traditional indemnity insurance.

As the insurance industry came to recognize that traditional indemnity insurance was losing market share to prepaid health plans, it responded by investing in many forms of managed care, including HMOs, PPOs, and exclusive provider organizations (EPOs). (EPOs are similar to PPOs in their organization, but they limit their beneficiaries to participating providers for health care services and pay no benefits for care delivered outside the network.) When, in the 1980s, major consolidations took place in the HMO industry, insurers seized the opportunity to buy a number of HMO plans. Since then, the insurance industry has played a significant role in the shaping of managed care.

An Expanding Market

The rapid growth of managed care reflects the recognition by employers and insurers that ways must be found to reduce costs while assuring that patients get appropriate care. Insurers increasingly see that unmanaged fee-for-service indemnity plans do not have mechanisms necessary to contain costs. As a consequence, many insurers have made major commitments to develop and maintain comprehensive managed care systems.

National HMO firms (defined as firms operating HMOs in two or more states, including commercial insurance companies that meet this criterion), along with Blue Cross/Blue Shield plans, will continue to account for nearly two-thirds of all HMOs and represent an overwhelming majority of Americans who are enrolled in managed care plans.[11]

By 1992, more than two-thirds of the total enrollment in the managed care plans of commercial insurers was in PPOs. Insurer-sponsored PPO enrollment increased 37 percent since 1988, from 13 million to approximately 17.8 million enrollees.[12] Of the approximately 8.3 million enrolled in insurer-sponsored HMOs, 67 percent were enrolled in IPA plans, 22 percent in group-model plans, and 9 percent in staff-model HMOs.[13] For further explication of these HMO models, see Chapter 3.

Blue Cross/Blue Shield plans also have seen a dramatic shift to managed care in the past decade. Blue Cross/Blue Shield has 68 independent plans that collectively insure 68 million members in the United States. The Blue Cross/Blue Shield Association reported that in 1992 31 percent of its membership was enrolled in a managed care plan, a dramatic change from the 1.5 percent enrolled in managed care in 1981. The association predicts that managed care enrollment will climb to 50 percent by the middle of the decade and reach 80 percent by the end of the decade.[14]

Change in Emphasis, Products, and Systems

Managed care has transformed the insurance industry. Instead of serving only as claims payers and underwriters (those who determine on what basis to accept an application for insurance), commercial health insurers are now managing both the delivery and financing of health benefits to beneficiaries.[15]

Managed care has required insurers to make substantial investments in physical and human capital as well as changes in many longstanding business practices. They are investing heavily in programs and products designed to increase the efficiency of the managed care products they offer. They now operate large HMO and PPO networks, POS plan options, and "integrated multiple options" that combine HMOs, indemnity plans, or PPOs in various ways.

Through joint ventures and multiple-insurer sponsorships, many medium-sized insurers are renting networks of providers. They are marketing utilization management programs that can be applied across all product lines, including traditional indemnity arrangements. Many are applying principles of managed care, such as hospital and outpatient precertification, to their traditional indemnity products. Precertification is the process whereby providers notify the insurer before nonemergency hospitalization of a patient. The insurer then approves payment for treatment or recommends an alternate course of action. Insurers may also require preauthorization or other screening processes to evaluate the need for expensive or invasive medical treatment delivered outside the hospital.

The insurers who have thrived in the managed care market are those who have collaborated effectively with the medical community and have integrated medical management, provider relations, and member service systems efficiently into their organizations.

■ The Current Managed Care Marketplace

The growth of managed care has accelerated significantly in the past five years, and an increasing proportion of consumers, providers, and payers are now participating in managed care. By 1991, an HIAA survey showed that for the first time a majority of the 150 million enrollees in employer-sponsored health plans belonged to a managed care plan.[16] By 1993, another survey also reported only 48 percent of employees were enrolled in traditional indemnity plans. (Figure 2.3)

The role of insurers in managed care has increased dramatically as well. Insurers now own or manage 43 percent of all HMOs.[17] In 1991, 33 percent of employees enrolled in PPOs were in plans administered by Blue Cross/Blue Shield,

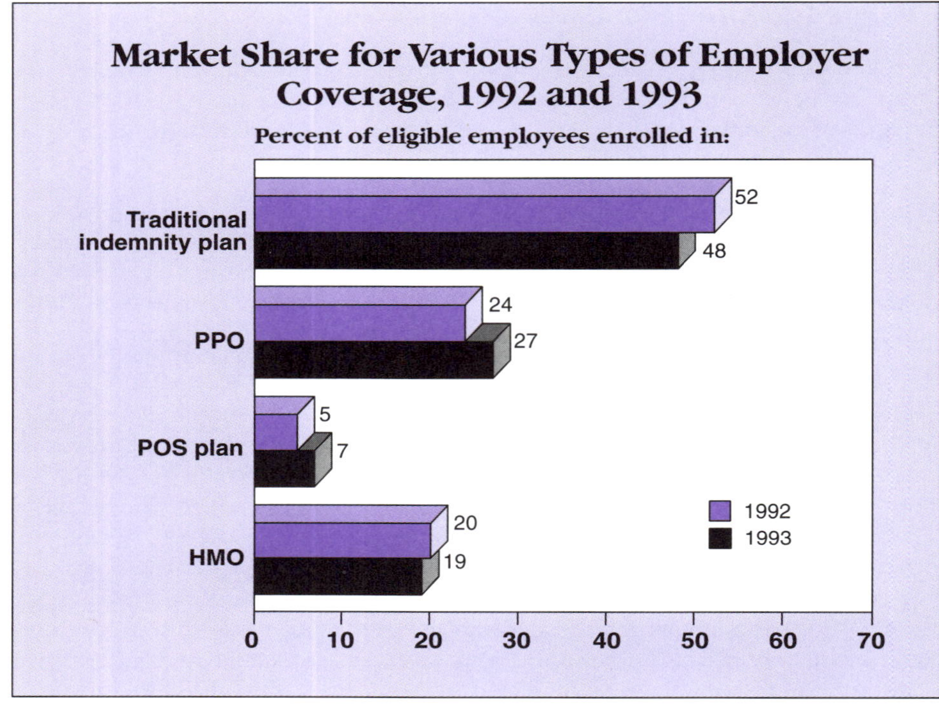

Figure 2.3

SOURCE: Foster Higgins National Survey of Employer-Sponsored Health Plans, 1993.

29 percent were in plans administered by a third-party administrator, and 28 percent were in PPO plans administered by a commercial insurer. Just 13 years ago, less than 1 percent of commercial health insurers' business was in managed care.[18]

These trends also have had a major impact on health care providers, because virtually all have had contact with managed care in some form, many through formal agreements. By 1993, more than 90 percent of the hospitals in the United States had some type of contract with one or more managed care organizations, and 75 percent of physicians in active practice had a contract with at least one.[19]

Another trend that is evolving is the managed care arrangement that addresses certain specialty care health services. One area where this is occurring is mental health. Behavioral health, also called mental health, has come under intense scrutiny within the past few years as employers, insurers, and society all struggle with the increasing demand for such services and the difficulty in managing costs for long-term treatment. Utilization of mental health and substance abuse care has increased in recent years, and costs for such services have grown at a proportionately greater rate than costs for primary care (routine medical care). For example, from 1987 to 1988, mental health costs to employers rose 27 percent, while employers' overall medical costs rose by 19 percent.[20] Insurers and employers have begun using managed care techniques to control the costs of behavioral health programs through specialty managed care arrangements. Often, such arrangements are called single-service HMOs, or single-service PPOs.

The cost of prescription drugs has been growing rapidly. Throughout the 1980s, the rate of increase in prescription drug costs exceeded the rate of increase in both the Consumer Price Index and the medical component of the Consumer Price Index.[21] In a staff report of The Special Committee on Aging to the United States Senate in September 1991, 6 percent of total health costs were attributed to prescription pharmaceuticals.[22] A study released by the General Accounting Office (GAO) in the summer of 1992 showed similar results, reporting that prices for some of the most widely used prescription drugs increased at nearly twice the overall health care inflation rate from 1986 to 1991.[23] In the case of prescription drugs, various cost control techniques are being developed by employers, insurers, and managed care companies. Drug utilization review, the use of defined pharmacy networks, and filling prescriptions through mail order are three techniques frequently used.

Desire for cost controls also has spawned a variety of managed care options in dental services. Employers, insurers, and HMOs have all sought to incorporate managed care techniques into special dental care plans.

Regional Variation in Enrollment

Managed care has penetrated some regions of the United States more deeply than others. (Figures 2.4 and 2.5) While total HMO enrollment has increased from 14 million to more than 45 million since 1984 and the number of individuals with access to PPOs has grown from 8 million to 35 million during the same period, much of this growth has taken place in fewer than 20 states. Variations from state to state can be considerable. For example, in 12 states, more than 20 percent of the population is enrolled in HMOs, while in other states less than 8 percent of the population are HMO enrollees.[24]

In 1992, HMO enrollment was greatest in the West (27 percent) and Northeast (20 percent), moderate in the Midwest (15 percent), and lowest in the South (9 percent).[25] California enrolled a higher proportion of its population in HMOs

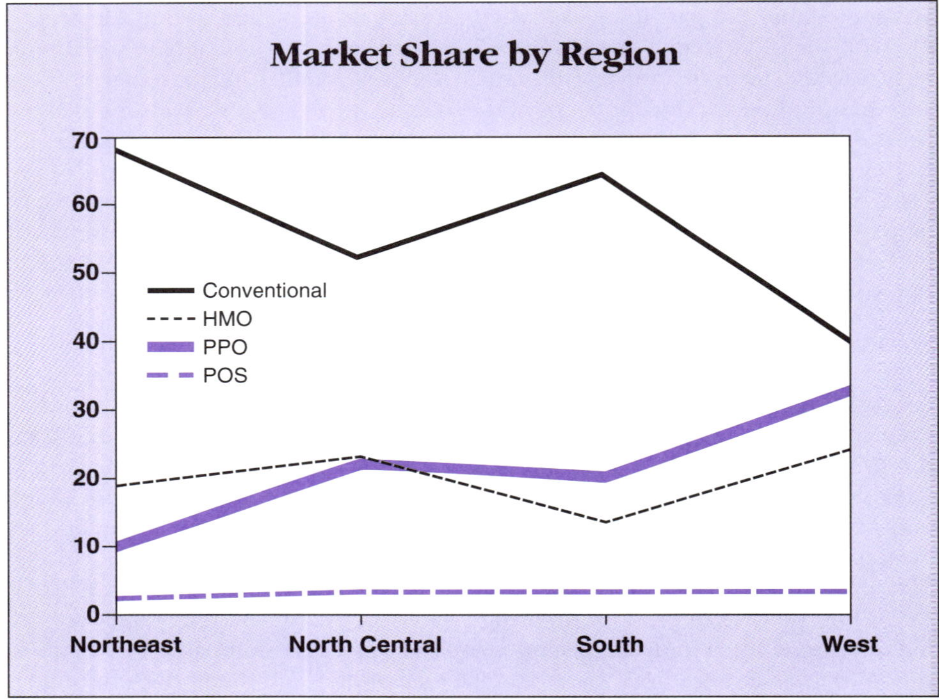

Figure 2.4

SOURCE: HIAA Employer Survey, 1992.

than any other state (35 percent), followed by Massachusetts (34.1 percent), Arizona (32.9 percent), Maryland (32.0 percent), Oregon (31 percent), and Minnesota (30.1 percent).[26] California, followed by Texas, enrolled more of its population in PPO plans than did any other state. Minnesota leads the nation in POS plan enrollment.

There is no doubt that differences in demographics and social and political development in the states have played a part in determining relative receptivity to managed care. In general, though, managed care has flourished in those areas in which it made an early, effective appearance.

Some cities have experienced managed care penetration rates so high that a managed care culture is said to exist. Minneapolis-St. Paul is a case in point. Managed care initiatives took hold early in Minnesota, whose demographic characteristics and populist traditions made it extremely receptive to experiments

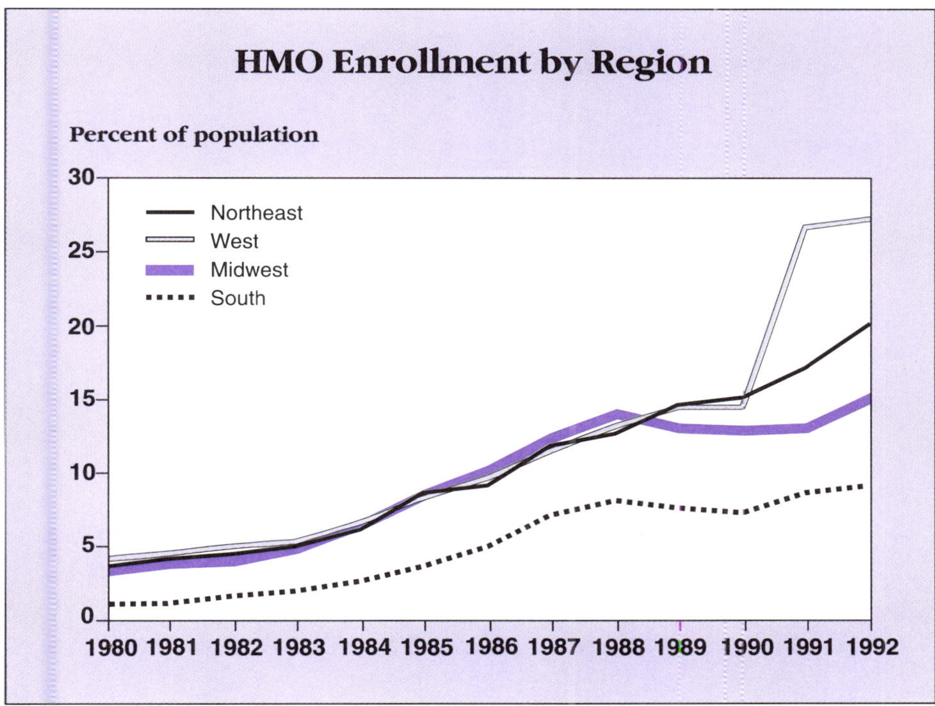

Figure 2.5

SOURCE: The InterStudy Competitive Edge, 1991, 1993.

in cooperative health care. By 1993, 46 percent of the population of the Twin Cities was enrolled in HMOs.[27] Rochester, New York, Worchester, Massachusetts, and San Francisco, California, were higher, however, with 54 percent, 51 percent, and 49 percent, respectively, of their populations enrolled. Managed care has developed into a mature and sophisticated product in these cities, and their experience illustrates the enormous potential for its development.

Although significant differences continue to exist among states in their involvement in managed care, these differences are shrinking. In 1980, there were 10 or more HMOs in only 10 states and only California had more than 1 million HMO enrollees. By 1993, 21 states had 10 or more HMOs, and 12 had HMO enrollments of more than 1 million.[28] The southern states have responded more slowly to innovative methods of health care organization, but HMO enrollment is growing steadily in this region, particularly in the South Atlantic region.

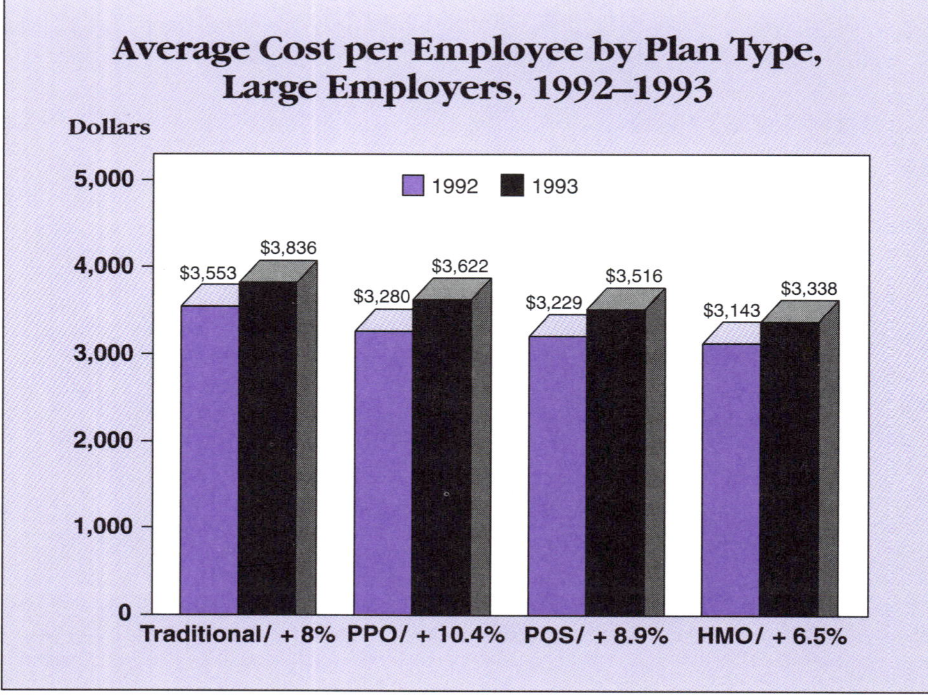

Figure 2.6

SOURCE: Foster Higgins National Survey of Employer-Sponsored Health Plans, 1993.

The Rural United States

The 23 percent of the nation's population that lives in rural areas presents special challenges for the delivery and financing of health care. Because this population is widely scattered and has a higher percentage of poor people than urban areas, it has not been able to attract and sustain large numbers of physicians and medical facilities. Thus, many rural areas suffer from limited access to health care.

Though rural populations could benefit from managed care's rational organization of delivery and financing, the absence of significant health care resources and lack of opportunities for competition between providers have been major impediments to the development of managed care networks in rural areas. De-

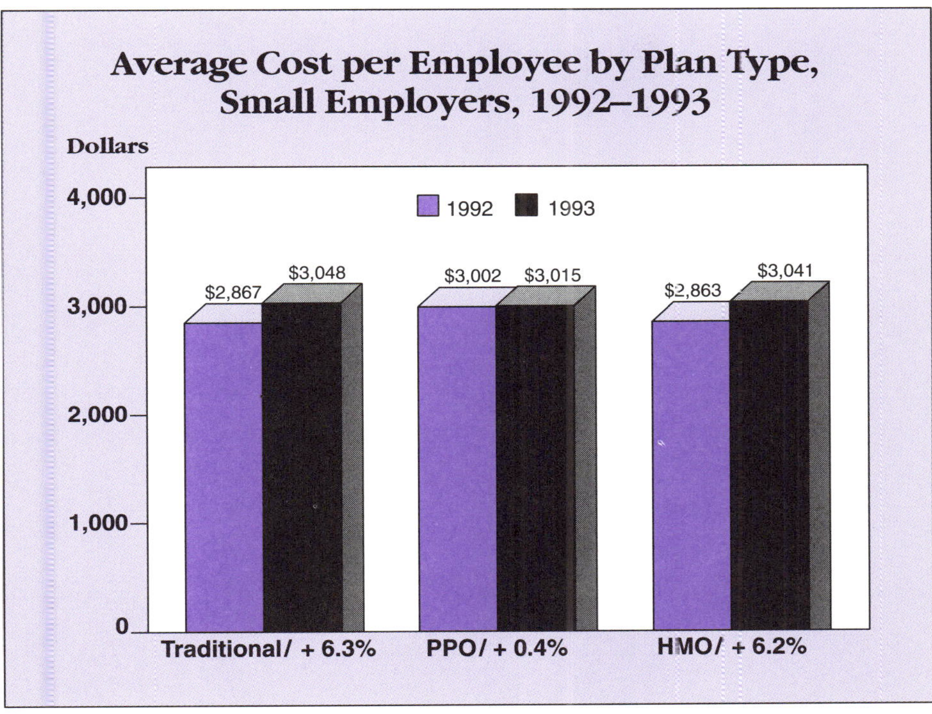

Figure 2.7

SOURCE: Foster Higgins National Survey of Employer-Sponsored Health Plans, 1993.

spite these problems, there has been some experimentation with adapting managed care concepts to rural areas.

It is interesting to note that some of the first managed care plans were created to solve access problems in remote areas. Managed care has the potential to solve such problems in rural areas now and in the future. A recent report,[29] commissioned by the National Rural Electric Cooperative Association and the Metropolitan Life Insurance Company, analyzed the operations of three PPOs and a staff-model HMO whose total operations serve 11 states. The report concluded that managed care is not only viable in rural areas but is growing. From this report, we know that of the rural employers who have measured their savings from managed care plans, most find that they are saving between 10 and 15 percent of usual and customary charges.

Percentage of Employees in Health Plans Offering Specified Covered Benefits, 1988 – 1993

	HMO 1988	HMO 1993	FFS 1988	FFS 1993	PPO 1988	PPO 1993
Adult physicals	96%	93%	20%	43%	37%	51%
Well-baby care	95	91	38	56	58	72
Outpatient mental health	92	90	93	94	95	96
Inpatient mental health	92	86	94	96	96	96
Substance abuse	93	90	84	91	91	93

Figure 2.8

SOURCES: KPMG Peat Marwick 1993 Survey of Employer-Sponsored Health Benefits; HIAA 1988 Health Benefits Study.

Measures of Effectiveness

Because of rapid growth and evolution, there is insufficient evidence to prove the effectiveness of managed care, especially with regard to the newer models of managed care. The impact of the different models on health care use, expenditures, and quality of care takes time to evaluate. However, some early results are significant. For example, a comparison of employee health costs by A. Foster Higgins demonstrates that costs for managed care enrollees were less than for those in conventional plans. (Figures 2.6 and 2.7)

These more favorable cost levels exist despite the fact that managed care generally offers a richer benefit package than do fee-for-service plans. (Figure 2.8) Both HMOs and PPOs maintained or improved the comprehensiveness of covered benefits during the period 1988–1993.

■ Summary

Managed care arose from the unique challenge of delivering and financing health care within the framework of the developing economic, political, and social environment of the United States. The forerunners of managed care emerged with the establishment of early prepaid group practices which began to build on the financing structure of health care benefits provided by employers. Federal support of managed care through the HMO Act in 1973, coupled with significant employer interest in managed care approaches to deal with rapidly rising costs, has produced significant HMO growth from the 1970s to present.

Corporate entrants, including insurers, have been important factors affecting managed care development. Insurers, recognizing the changing marketplace, responded by investing in many forms of managed care programs with many types of organizational relationships to increase efficiency and assure quality.

Managed care, with significant regional variation in market penetration, continues to grow and expand, affecting even rural areas.

■ Key Terms

American Medical Association (AMA)
Baylor Plan
Behavioral health
Blue Cross/Blue Shield
Capital markets
Certification
Coinsurance
Collective bargaining
Consumer Price Index
Copayment
Coverage
Deductible
Demography
Exclusive Provider Organizations (EPOs)
Federally qualified
Fee-for-service discounts
Fee-for-service medicine
Gatekeepers

General Accounting Office (GAO)
Group medical catastrophe coverage
Group-model HMO
Health Maintenance Organization (HMO)
HMO Act
Hospital bill audit
Hospitalization
Individual Practice Association (IPA)
Integrated multiple options
Managed mental health
Managed pharmacy programs
Medical management
Medical service bureau

Medical societies
Multispecialty group practice
Mutual benefit society
National Association of Insurance Commissioners (NAIC)
Network providers
Open-ended HMO
Out-of-plan care
Physician associations
Physician peer review
Point-of-Service (POS) Plans
Precertification
Preferred Provider Organization (PPO)
Premiums

Prepaid group practices
Prepayment
Primary care
Prospective screening
Providers
Risk
Second surgical opinions
Selective provider
  relationships
Sherman Antitrust Act
Solo practitioners
Specialty managed care
  arrangements
Staff-model plans
Third-party vendors
Traditional indemnity
  insurance
Underwriters
Utilization
Utilization controls
Utilization review
Voluntary certification
  process
Wrap-around coverage

Chapter 3

ORGANIZATION OF MANAGED CARE ARRANGEMENTS

33 *Introduction*

34 *Health Maintenance Organizations*

52 *Factors That Affect Managed Care*

53 *Summary*

53 *Key Terms*

■ Introduction

Many types of managed care arrangements have evolved over time, and variations continue to evolve. The United States, which has a private, competitive model of health insurance, has been more innovative in developing models of health care financing and delivery than those countries with government-controlled health insurance programs.

Though managed care continues to evolve, there are several key factors common to all arrangements. These include:

- management of both the financing and delivery of health care;

- institution of cost control techniques;

- some sharing of financial risk between providers and payers, and

- management of the utilization of services.

There is a continuum of managed care models that moves from the least control by the managed care organization to the most control. The least controlled programs, such as traditional indemnity insurance with managed care features, allow unlimited access to providers, but at higher cost to the payer and the enrollee. Programs with the most control, such as the staff-model HMO (see below), strictly limit access to providers, but at lower cost to payers and enrollees.

As managed care becomes more sophisticated in its approaches, practitioners are being asked to provide the highest quality of care for the most reasonable cost. The competitive health care marketplace in the United States creates an ever-changing managed care environment in the struggle to reach this goal.

It should be remembered that at present, no managed care model can offer high levels of benefits, unlimited access to providers, and low cost at the same time. The best any managed care plan can expect to accomplish is two of these three features. Some plans will stress cost and access, while others will stress benefits and cost, or access and benefits.

■ Health Maintenance Organizations

Health Maintenance Organizations (HMOs) are the most sophisticated of current managed care arrangements in their efforts to control cost, utilization, and access. In general, HMOs have the following common characteristics:

- They offer a comprehensive set of health benefits, usually on a fixed-premium basis, to a voluntarily enrolled population.

- The choice of providers is usually limited to the HMO's network of physicians and hospitals.

- They limit or eliminate out-of-pocket expenses to the enrollee, as long as enrollees seek care from HMO-designated providers.

- They use the primary care physician as a gatekeeper or manager of referrals for specialty care or hospitalization.

Some HMOs operate as a separate line of business within an insurance company; others operate independently and are not affiliated with an insurer. In contrast to traditional insurance arrangements, the HMO provides services directly to its enrollees either by employing or by contracting with physicians and hospitals. When recruited to join HMOs, physician providers undergo a credentialing process, involving a careful review of educational qualifications, work history, status of hospital privileges and malpractice history and, sometimes, an interview with a peer review committee. The scrutiny provides the basis for selecting a specified number and type of providers that make up a network.

Payment for Services

In an HMO, enrollees or employers pay a fixed monthly or annual premium for the full range of services offered rather than the fee-for-service approach of traditional indemnity insurance. The HMO assumes the risk that the costs for providing care will not exceed those premiums. The idea is to encourage efficiency and provide services designed to keep members healthy.

At present, there are four major HMO models; they differ according to the ways in which they contract with and reimburse providers. They are the staff model, the group model, the individual practice association, and the network or mixed model.

The Staff-Model HMO

The staff-model HMO frequently owns the clinical facilities used by patients enrolled in the HMO. The physicians providing service are directly employed by the HMO. These physicians provide service only to patients enrolled in the HMO plan. This method of employing physicians for the exclusive use by HMO plan enrollees is called a closed panel and offers the tightest control over the practice patterns of physicians, thus allowing more control over utilization of services. These physicians receive salaries and may also receive incentive payments or bonuses based on performance, but the HMO is at financial risk for the cost of services.

Advantages and disadvantages. Staff-model HMOs may be the most convenient for enrollees because most of them offer complete ambulatory care services such as physicians' offices, laboratory, x-ray, and pharmacy services in one centralized location. However, this aspect of staff-model HMOs can make start-up and implementation very expensive. Thus, the staff-model HMO requires considerably more up-front capital than other HMO models.

The Group-Model HMO

Unlike the staff-model HMO, the group-model HMO contracts with a multispecialty group to provide care to plan members. The physicians are not employees of the HMO, but actually are employed by the group practice. In some cases, the HMO actually forms the group practice to care for the HMO's members, but the group practice maintains its own separate corporate identity. In some instances, the group practice may own the HMO.

Physicians in the group-model practice in facilities owned by the group or by the HMO. The group is generally paid a fixed amount for each individual enrolled in the HMO. This amount covers the cost of all primary and referral care. This payment (called capitation) is made in advance as opposed to for each service provided. In some cases, physician practice groups may contract with the HMO on a cost basis to provide services. The payment is made based on costs, rather than a set fee. Depending on the group-model arrangement, some groups may be allowed to provide service to patients outside the HMO and bill those patients separately. Some group practices also are at risk for all, or a portion of, hospital care in capitated rates paid by the HMO.

Staff-model and group-model HMOs are called closed-panel HMOs. The term "closed-panel" refers to the fact that the HMO contracts with physicians on an exclusive basis to provide health services solely to the enrollees of the plan. Nonplan physicians are excluded from participation.

Advantages and disadvantages.   One major advantage of the group model over the staff model is that the group model may offer lower capital costs to the HMO. There is less need to purchase medical facilities, and the cost of capitation is often less than the physician salaries in the staff model.

The group model may be at a disadvantage compared to other models because of fewer ambulatory care sites or less well distributed sites available to members. Also, this model, while still offering a significant ability to control practice patterns and utilization, does not offer as much control as the staff model, where physicians are employees of the HMO.

Individual or Independent Practice Association

In this model, the HMO contracts with physicians in private practice either individually or in organized groups. A majority of HMOs are organized in this way. The Individual or Independent Practice Association (IPA) is a separate legal entity that contracts with the HMO. Its physicians retain their independent practices and their own offices. IPA physicians continue in private practice, but they see HMO patients as a part of that practice. Participation in the IPA is open to physicians in the community.

Most HMOs compensate IPAs through use of primary care capitation arrangements. The IPA receives a capitated amount for each enrollee from the HMO. This payment covers primary care services. In some cases, the capitation payment goes directly to the physician. In others, the IPA reimburses its participating primary care physicians on a fee-for-service basis or a combination of fee-for-service and capitation.

When fee-for-service is the method of reimbursement, frequently a portion of the payment is withheld, as a method of risk sharing. If services are delivered cost-effectively, the amount withheld is distributed to the providers that are involved in the withhold arrangements. Most specialty physicians are reimbursed on a "discounted fee-for-service with withhold" basis. Generally, enrollees in HMOs can seek care from specialists only if they are referred by a primary care physician. In some IPAs, primary care physicians are at financial risk for referral to specialty care and hospitals. This can be done through a variety of risk arrangements.

Stop-loss arrangements.   Most withhold arrangements include a stop-loss arrangement to protect physicians from suffering severe financial loss if a few patients have catastrophic medical costs. Stop-loss is a type of insurance that provides protection from claims that are greater than a specific dollar amount per covered person. Stop-loss is a common protection against financial loss from catastrophic cases.

There are many different types of stop-loss arrangements. Most stop-loss arrangements predetermine liability limits on an aggregate or specific basis.

Aggregate stop-loss insurance will reimburse the buyer for claims that exceed an aggregate limit within a specified time period. The limit is usually set at a percentage of expected claims (for example, 125 percent) and is expressed as a monthly amount multiplied by the number of insureds. Factors involved in establishing the limit as a percentage of expected claims include the number of covered individuals, claim frequency, and average size of claim.

Specific stop-loss insurance will provide protection against large individual claims by limiting the buyer's liability for any one insured person during a specified time period. The specific stop-loss limit usually will be expressed as a dollar amount, such as $10,000.

Physician-hospital organizations as a form of IPA.   Physician-hospital organizations (PHOs) are an increasingly common IPA group practice arrangement that occurs when hospitals and physicians organize for purposes of contracting with managed care organizations. These relationships are formally organized, contractual or corporate in character, and can include physicians who are not members of a hospital's medical staff.

A PHO is a legal entity formed and owned by one or more hospitals and physician groups in order to obtain payer contracts and to further mutual interests. The physicians maintain ownership of their practices while agreeing to accept managed care patients under the terms of the PHO agreement. The PHO serves as a negotiating, contracting, and marketing unit.

PHO relationships are essentially symbiotic—hospitals have to have the capital and organizational infrastructure that physicians often lack. The hospital, on the other hand, is vulnerable to the changing marketplace because of its physical and structural commitment to its service area. The PHO enables physicians to focus on medicine and clinical management issues while the hospital serves as the administrative or financial center.

PHOs are constructed in many different ways and with commonly shared organizational features. A typical PHO provides for equal physician and hospital ownership and equal board representation. The physicians may first organize an

IPA, which appoints representatives to the PHO board, often requiring a quorum of equal numbers of physicians and hospital representatives to vote. PHOs may vary in the degree to which they engage in risk contracting and the care with which they evaluate physicians during the selection process. However, once they are organized, they may contract with IPA-HMOs or other managed care arrangements discussed below.

The various PHO structures include:

- **Physician-Hospital Organization.** (See definition above).

- **Management Services Organization (MSO).** MSOs are legal entities formed to provide administrative and practice management services to individual physicians or group practices. The MSO can be one of the least integrated forms of physician-hospital alliance because it is connected to physicians only through an administrative services contract. In its more formal structure, an MSO can provide an avenue for shared equity ownership with the physicians. In addition, many MSOs buy the practice assets of their physicians. MSOs can take many forms—some are direct hospital subsidiaries, while others are free-standing and may be owned by investors.

- **Group Practice Without Walls.** A group practice without walls is a network of physicians who have merged into one legal entity, but continue to practice independently in their own office locations. This model maintains the autonomy of physician practice style while affording physicians the benefits of centralized administrative services, economies of scale, new marketing opportunities, and additional legal protection. The relationship of the hospital to such a group may vary.

- **Medical Foundation.** In the medical foundation model, a nonprofit foundation is established which purchases the business and clinical assets of a physician group or several independent physicians. The foundation provides all the business and administrative support services needed to support the practice. In California, which prohibits the corporate practice of medicine, the foundation model is popular because there is a special exemption for medical foundations that accept payment for physician services.

- **Integrated Delivery System.** The fully integrated model combines a full range of physician and other health services under one corporate entity. The system may include one or more hospitals, group practices, health plans, and other health care operations. Physicians are either employees of the system or members of an affiliated group.

The PHO seeks ways to control the cost of hospital and specialty services by attempting to secure its physician referral base and maintain control over physicians' ambulatory care business. It also serves to cut costs, control utilization, and document and improve quality of care.

PHOs vary across many dimensions, such as:

- the degree of capitalization;
- types of administrative and clinical management functions;
- composition of the membership between primary care and specialists; and
- goals of the organization.

Advantages and disadvantages of IPAs. The IPA model has several distinct advantages. There are fewer start-up costs and ongoing capital outlays needed from the HMO, because the HMO does not need to own facilities or pay salaries. Also, IPAs can offer members a wider choice of physicians, which makes them more appealing and is probably a significant factor in the growth of this model in recent years.

The major disadvantage of the IPA is that it offers the least control of any of the HMO arrangements. Because IPA physicians retain their private practices, they do not have the same sense of belonging to an HMO as do staff- and group-model physicians. It is more difficult to control practice patterns and utilization of health services with this more individualized form of managed care.

For the PHO-IPA arrangement, advantages include low initial capitalization requirements, the provision of a forum for improved physician-hospital communications, and the potential for developing stronger mutual interests between the hospital and its physicians. However, a major reason for the growth of PHOs is that they are politically manageable, enabling the hospital and physicians to share the decision-making power more equitably, with limited risk to each party.

Network- or Mixed-Model HMO

Network-model HMOs, sometimes referred to as mixed-model HMOs, are provider arrangements that contract with a number of IPAs or group practices to provide physician services to HMO enrollees. This model is a multiple provider arrangement consisting of group, staff, or IPA structures in combination. Sometimes, a network model will contract with a number of small primary physician groups and will reimburse them on a capitated basis. These groups are then responsible for providing compensation to member physicians. In other cases, the network-model HMO may contract with primary care and specialty care groups as well as hospitals. This more integrated HMO helps to reduce risk to primary care physician groups in regard to utilization by spreading the risk to other provider groups. Network models may be either closed or open panels.

Advantages and disadvantages. The major advantage of the network model is that it can offer the broadest provider participation of any HMO. This has appeal for many prospective HMO enrollees. However, physician participation varies from market to market and plan to plan and is dependent on a number of factors. Although the network model may be structured to accommodate broader participation by allowing individual practitioners and groups equal participation, in reality, the IPA model could have equal or greater participation.

The negative aspects of the network model can be similar to those of the IPA or group model. The effectiveness of controls of utilization can vary, depending on the types of contract arrangements in this model.

Preferred Provider Organizations

A Preferred Provider Organization (PPO) is a managed care arrangement consisting of a group of hospitals, physicians, and other providers who have contracts with an insurer, employer, third-party administrator, or other sponsoring group to provide health care services to covered persons. Most PPOs provide a comprehensive set of health benefits and, usually, a full range of health services. Some PPOs, however, focus on a single service. These newer arrangements consist of groups of providers assembled to offer specialty services. One of the most common single-service arrangements is a mental health PPO.

Provider participation in the PPO is determined by a selection process, and PPOs often limit the size of the network of participating providers. Unlike HMOs, PPOs allow participants to use primary care providers outside the PPO. However, the enrollee has a financial incentive to seek services from a participating provider because of higher copayments, coinsurance (percentage of incurred medical expenses that the patient must pay), or deductibles outside the network.

Common Elements of PPOs

Most PPOs incorporate the following operational elements:

- Limitations on the Number of Providers: In the PPO, a sponsoring organization (often an insurer) contracts with a finite set of providers who meet specified criteria. Criteria can include cost-efficiency, scope of service, or credentials.

- Negotiated Payments: The primary care physicians (and, in some cases, all providers) in the PPO network agree to accept a negotiated level of reimbursement.

- Utilization Review: Participating physicians agree to follow the utilization review procedures administered by the PPO.

Reimbursement Mechanisms

The financial advantages to PPO providers may result from an increased volume of patients, more rapid reimbursement, and reductions in uncollected or uncollectible accounts. In some cases, primary care physicians act as gatekeepers by assuming the responsibility for managing referrals to specialists and referring patients exclusively to other PPO-contracted providers and admitting patients only to hospitals with PPO contracts.

In a gatekeeper model PPO, in order to receive benefits for specialty services, PPO patients must first seek care from their primary care physician. This function helps to control high-cost specialty services. Patients are discouraged from self-referral to specialty services because low or no benefits will be provided. They are encouraged to seek primary care first, and their health needs may be met by the primary care physician without more costly specialty care.

PPO providers are most often reimbursed on a discounted fee-for-service basis, although a few are capitated for primary care services. PPOs rarely have risk arrangements that include withholds for specialty care because of the relatively loose control of out-of-network specialty care. Some states have laws that prohibit PPOs from capitating physician services and allow only HMOs to do so. A few states prohibit PPOs from using other types of risk arrangements (such as withholds) as well.

Advantages and disadvantages. There are several advantages to PPO arrangements. Among them are:

- providing greater choice by allowing patients to use either a participating provider or a non-network provider for care;

- using some of the techniques of managed care such as utilization review and case management to control costs and monitor quality; and

- providing quick reimbursement and an increased volume of patients in exchange for lower negotiated fees.

Among the disadvantages of PPOs is that the quality assurance mechanisms in the PPO are less extensive than in the HMO because of differences in organizational structure. PPOs have less control over provider behavior, and data collection can be less comprehensive than in other managed care entities, particularly HMOs. The PPO can be less rigorous in its utilization review and less demanding of its providers in the area of cost containment, particularly if there is no gatekeeper or other type of risk sharing. Many feel that financial incentives are the best mechanisms for controlling costs.

The Exclusive Provider Organization

The Exclusive Provider Organization (EPO) has its roots in the PPO primarily because it is an arrangement consisting of a group of providers who have contractual arrangements with an insurer, employer, third-party administrator, or other sponsoring group. The EPO represents a more restrictive, tightly controlled PPO. Although the criteria for provider participation may be the same as those in the PPO, many EPOs have a more restrictive provider selection and credentialing process. Consequently, many EPO networks have a smaller pool of more thoroughly reviewed physicians; thus, patients have access to higher-quality providers but have a narrower range of choice. In the EPO, the enrollee must seek services exclusively (hence the name Exclusive Provider Organization) from participating providers in order to be eligible for benefits. As in an HMO, patients enrolled in an EPO must receive their care from network providers or pay the entire cost themselves.

The EPO contracts with a set of providers who meet specified credentialing criteria. As in the PPO, the provider agrees to accept the negotiated level of reimbursement, follow prescribed utilization review procedures, refer to other EPO-contracted providers, and have patients admitted only to network hospitals. Providers are generally reimbursed on a discounted fee-for-service basis. EPOs may have provider risk arrangements that include withholds or other type of incentive payment provision, but most contracts do not contain such incentives.

Advantages and disadvantages. EPOs are frequently started by employers to save on health care costs. They are used as replacements for traditional indemnity plans and emulate many of the positive features of HMOs. However, because of the severe restrictions on the choice of health care providers with no alternatives, many of these plans are not viewed favorably by employees. Large employers rarely choose to use the EPO as the sole replacement for traditional indemnity insurance, preferring to offer the EPO as one option among several.

Point-of-Service Plans

Point-of-Service (POS) plans, a relatively new model of managed care, are one of the fastest-growing options. POS plans combine features of the HMO and PPO. They provide a comprehensive set of health benefits and offer a full range of health services, much the same as the HMO. However, the members do not have to choose how to receive services until they need them. Members can then opt to use the defined managed care program and the network or go out-of-plan for services but pay the difference for nonplan benefits (e.g., 100 percent coverage for in-plan care vs. 80 percent coverage out-of-plan). Common characteristics of POS plans include:

- using the primary care physician in a gatekeeper role to control specialist referrals;

- allowing the enrollee/insured to use out-of-network providers but at a reduced level of benefits (generally in the form of higher copayments); the enrollee who opts out of the network must file claims; and

- allowing enrollees to seek care in or out of the network at each point of service or each time they seek care.

The POS plan that uses the HMO network usually has contracting arrangements similar to those of the HMO. There may be additional risk-sharing arrangements with providers for out-of-network care, although some states have regulations against such arrangements.

Less common is the PPO-type POS plan that uses the traditional discounted fee-for-service arrangement to reimburse providers. In this arrangement, providers do not share in the risk for out-of-network care. Financial incentives for providers are minimal and generally are in the form of utilization review. The enrollee also has a financial incentive to seek network care to avoid higher copayments.

Utilization management techniques in the POS are similar to those in the HMO. They may vary for enrollees who opt out of the network at the point of service but very few POS plans allow unrestricted fee-for-service care to be received outside the network.

The quality assurance activities within the network do not apply outside it because there is no selection process for the out-of-network provider. In addition, there is no contract obligating both parties to certain administrative procedures, and there is little or no intervention in the out-of-network provider's actions.

Advantages and disadvantages. POS plans provide many of the controls and important advantages of HMOs and PPOs while allowing the flexibility of out-of-network choice. Employers view POS plans as a positive way to move from exclusive use of traditional indemnity plans to managed care. The employer has the benefit of some of the cost-containment features of managed care, while maintaining flexibility for those employees who choose to pay more for provider choice.

In addition, many HMOs and insurance carriers with HMOs have found that adopting POS options in their plans have made them more attractive to employers and other purchasers of health insurance. Once people are enrolled in POS programs, they eventually become comfortable with the provider networks that are part of the program and use them most, if not all, of the time.

The negative aspect of the POS is the lack of control available to the insurer for out-of-network usage. Generally, it is felt that this lack of control prevents cost-containment techniques from achieving their full potential.

Preventive Care Benefits

HMO and POS plans typically cover routine care and preventive medicine programs at 100 percent or for only a minimal copayment. These benefits, which are generally not available in indemnity plans, are a benefit of managed care plans when a primary care physician is used to oversee patient care and make appropriate referrals to network specialists or other providers. In some PPO plans, such preventive and routine care benefits are available only if patients select network providers. Preventive care can help control overall health benefit costs, because enrollees who have those benefits are less likely to put off treatment until a condition becomes more serious and treatment more costly.

Limited Service Models or Specialty HMOs

As managed care has evolved, several areas of health care delivery have been singled out for individual management. Behavioral health, prescription drugs, and dental services are three areas often managed through single- or limited-service plans. Single-service HMOs and PPOs have developed in states where permitted. Employers, insurers, and other managed care plans contract for such services through the single-service HMO or PPO. These single-service entities are often called "carve-outs" because the area in which they offer special services is carved out of the standard benefit plan to be managed individually.

Many managed care organizations and traditional insurers have found it difficult to control costs in these areas of health care service. Therefore, new specialty care providers have organized themselves to respond to concerns about growing costs in these chronic care and longer-term treatment areas. Often, it is the specialty care provider who establishes the single-service management in these carve-outs. It is common for some single-service plans to accept financial risk through a capitation arrangement. In this way, the single-service plan functions much as the HMO.

Behavioral Health Programs

Behavioral or mental health services, as mentioned in Chapter 2, present some special problems in cost control for employers and insurers. Traditional indemnity insurers have implemented several approaches to control these costs:

- defining and setting limits on the hospital length of stay;

- limiting the total dollar amount of coverage;

- increasing copayment levels;

- increasing premiums; or

- substituting outpatient care or partial hospitalization (daytime hospital services only, with no overnight stay) for full inpatient stays.

An increase in utilization and costs for behavioral health and substance abuse services over the past decade prompted employers who provide health care protection to their workers to seek managed care strategies to contain these costs. As a result, mental health and substance abuse managed care specialty programs were some of the first to be carved out of health benefit plans by employers and insurers eager to restrain this fast growing health expenditure.

Today, employers, HMOs, and insurers contract with third-party mental health management vendors who have had success in managing and lowering the costs of these services. These managed care specialty programs make use of traditional managed care controls. For example, they may use:

- case management techniques;

- utilization monitoring to assess cost-effective alternatives to inpatient and residential care (e.g., partial hospitalization and home care);

- professional review of proposed services to determine the most cost-effective treatment;

- development of 24-hour availability and access to care;

- integration of managed behavioral health programs with employee assistance programs (EAPs) to provide a managed care environment rather than a patient referral program that can be costly;

- other data and quality management techniques such as guidelines and protocols, which will be discussed later in this course; and

- improved communication between network providers.

Although evaluation and performance criteria have at times been more slowly developed and more difficult to apply in behavioral health than in other areas of medicine, managed mental health programs still serve an increasing proportion of health benefit plans and employee assistance programs.

Prescription Drug Programs

Almost all group health benefit plans provide some coverage for prescription drugs. Data from the *1992 HIAA Employer Survey* suggest that more than 90 percent of HMOs, PPOs, and conventional plans offer prescription drug benefits.[30] With coverage so widespread, anything affecting the cost and flexibility of a prescription drug plan will have an effect on most health benefit plans.

With the explosion in costs and utilization of prescription drugs, and the attendant impact on health benefit plans, insurers and employers have introduced managed care techniques into prescription drug benefit plans.

Pharmacy management programs help to monitor and control the utilization and cost of prescription drugs. They may include group or bulk purchasing, the use of open or closed pharmacy networks, and drug utilization review, but the use of voluntary formularies is their most effective weapon against the escalation of drug costs. A formulary is a list of preferred pharmaceutical products to be used by a plan's network physicians. Formularies are based on evaluations of the efficacy, safety, and cost-effectiveness of drugs. Some formularies require generic substitutions for more expensive brand name drugs, while others provide information on lower-cost drugs that are therapeutic equivalents. (A generic drug is one that has the identical makeup as a brand name drug. A therapeutic equivalent is one that is not chemically identical, but produces similar results.)

Another important function of some pharmacy management programs is the collection and interpretation of information about the prescribing habits of physicians. This information is useful in managing physician networks and can be an important tool in persuading physicians to practice cost-effective, high-quality medicine. Similar profiling of drug use by patients is often beneficial as well, because keeping complete drug histories on individuals directly improves the quality of the information necessary to deliver optimum care.

Managed care pharmacy benefits generally include:

- prescriptions filled at designated (or network) pharmacies;
- physician adherence to drug formularies when prescribing drugs;
- higher out-of-pocket charges to patients for use of brand name drugs;
- limiting the pharmacy benefit to those drugs prescribed by network physicians only; and
- use of mail order pharmacies to fill prescriptions for chronic medications, taking advantage of packaging in bulk.

Dental Specialty Programs

Costs and cost containment are the primary stimuli for employers' interest in managed dental care. Benefit managers and insurers have begun to identify potential advantages of a managed care approach to dental benefits and are discovering whether benefit enhancements similar to those realized for medical services and expenses may emerge when applied to dental coverage.

These enhancements might include:

- greater cost-containment efficiencies;
- cost moderations for benefits;
- an increase in quality of dental care;
- standardization of quality care; and
- more dental benefits per unit of cost.

The *1992 HIAA Employer Survey* reported that 22 percent of employees in HMOs had dental benefits.[31] More than half of all payments for dental services are out-of-pocket for consumers. The remaining 44.4 percent is covered by private insurance.

Traditional dental insurance has commonly used fee-for-service reimbursement for dental care. Most indemnity insurance restricts the paid benefit to usual, customary, and reasonable fees, an annual benefit cap, and qualified claims. For dental benefits however, the trend away from unmanaged fee-for-service was noted in the *1988 HIAA Employer Survey*,[32] though most individuals who have private dental insurance have a fee-for-service arrangement. (Figure 3.1)

The movement toward managed dental care began with employees who had indemnity insurance; thus, many managed dental benefit plans are considered to be managed indemnity, based on fee-for-service reimbursement. The transition was easier because the changes were less disruptive or apparent to employees than other managed care options.

Managed indemnity benefits are characterized by:

- low provider selection restrictions; and
- utilization review and enhanced claims review by dental professionals.

Dental PPOs are very similar to fee-for-service indemnity plans but are characterized by a network of dental care providers. Dental networks are developed in much the same way as early PPO networks, where the primary criterion for network selection is the successful negotiation of fees. In many fee-for-service dental plans, patients' choices of a dental provider may be unrestricted, but provider selection may be influenced by financial incentives, such as low or no deductibles and/or copayments for using contracted providers. Typical PPOs may

- contract with providers by accepting lower-cost providers; and
- seek discounted fee arrangements or make use of fee schedules.

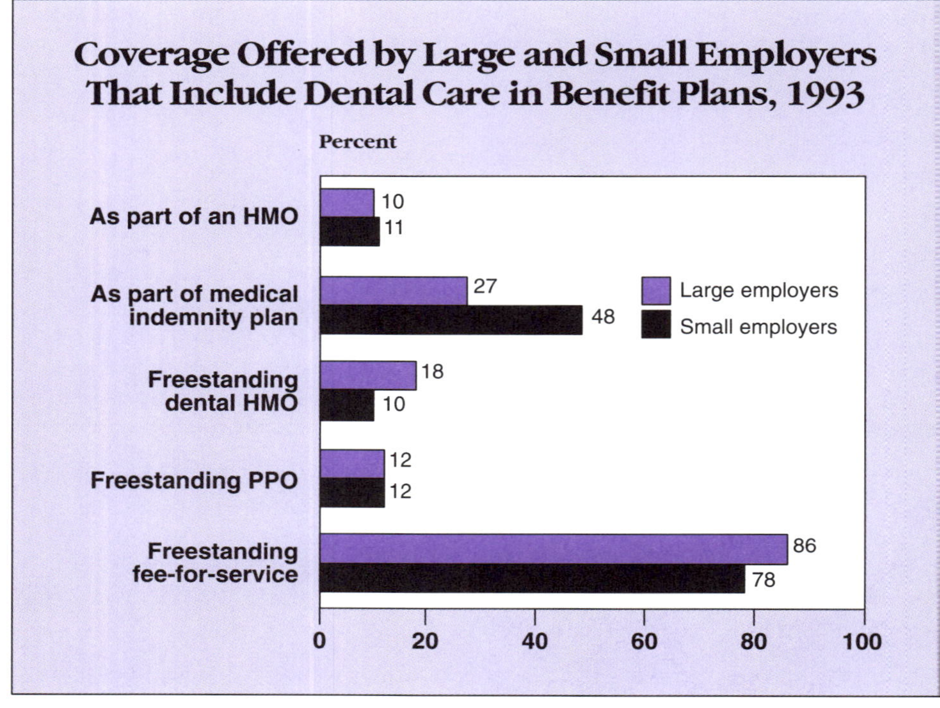

Figure 3.1

SOURCE: Foster Higgins National Survey of Employer-Sponsored Health Plans, 1993.
NOTE: Some employers offer more than one plan.

Most dental PPO enrollees enjoy a 10 to 20 percent cost saving over indemnity rates. Financial rewards to the plan and patients are expected to result from creating a healthy enrollee base, reduced expenditures for services, professional claims reviews, and utilization management.

Dental plans may be part of a broad medical service contract, supplementary to the medical contract and requiring additional premiums, or unbundled as a stand-alone or carved-out benefit under a separate contract. Some large HMOs are electing to contract for dental benefits with prepaid dental plans and/or PPOs rather than continue to manage the benefit themselves. Prepaid dental plans are capitated arrangements much like prepaid group practices. The *1992 HIAA Employers Survey* reported that 43 percent of employees enrolled in PPOs had dental benefits.[33]

Dental HMOs (DHMOs) use the same managed care techniques for dental benefits as other HMOs. For example, prepaid dental plans credential dental care providers for licensure and certification, review the history of professional disciplinary actions, and assure liability insurance coverage. Because of competitive pressures and liability concerns, the practice patterns of dental practitioners are periodically reviewed for consistency with the organizations' goals. They make use of professional claims review, review of utilization statistics, and reviews of office safety and infection control procedures.

The DHMO assumes the financial risk and responsibility for providing dental services to a specific population for a capitated payment per individual or family. DHMO ownership includes HMOs, hospitals, physicians, insurance companies, independent investors, and third-party administrators.

DHMOs may be staff, IPA (See Figure 3.2), or network models. As with other HMOs, staff models employ their own professional personnel. IPAs execute contracts with independent dentists, who may also continue in independent practice while using the IPA as a primary or supplemental source of income. In contrast, networks contract with one or more legal entities that represent professional practitioners as a united group. New point-of-service DHMOs allow insureds to opt out of the HMO at any time and to treat the benefit as an indemnity plan much the same as the medical POS.

Over the past three years, employers have begun unbundling dental benefits from their medical plans, as have some HMOs. This allows them to offer the benefit as a freestanding plan, allowing employees either to select the dental benefit or decline it for other alternatives in their employers' flexible benefit arrangements. (Figure 3.3)

In 1991, 86 percent of HMOs offered unbundled services to employers as a result of increasing popularity of this arrangement. Dental and prescription benefit plans were the most common carve-outs. These unbundled plans are entirely separate from HMOs' medical and medical-surgical coverage, and 38 percent of HMOs offer dental specialty programs as a part of these unbundled arrangements. The programs provide supplementary coverage for a dental benefit at an additional premium. Of the four HMO plan types below, the unbundled dental program was reported as follows:

- 15 percent among group plans;
- 16 percent among IPA models;
- 19 percent among network models; and
- 2 percent among staff models.

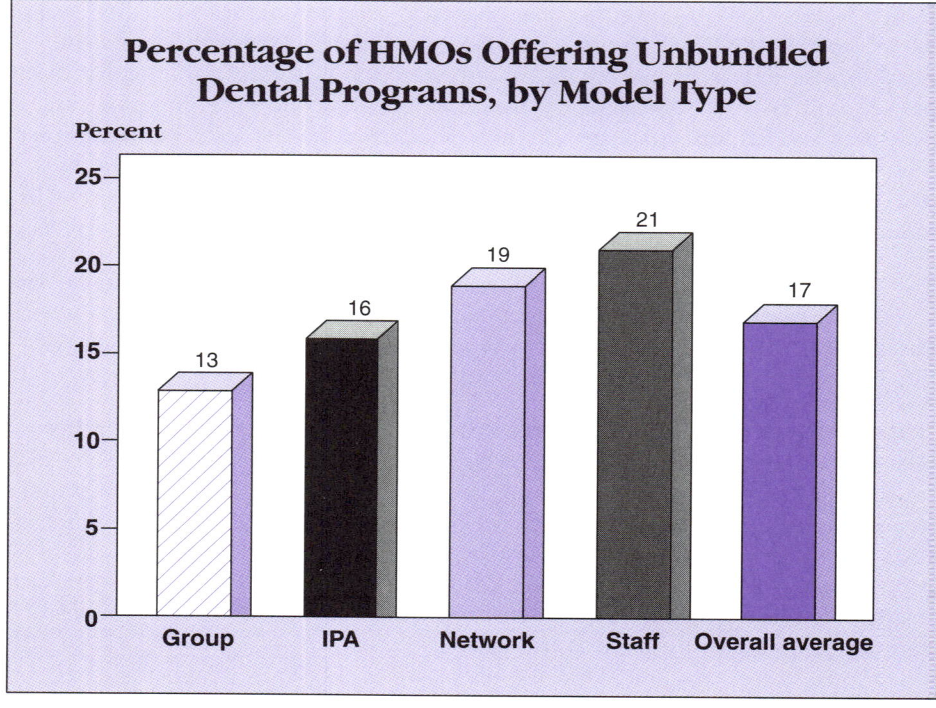

Figure 3.2

SOURCE: Marion Merrill Dow Managed Care Digest, HMO Edition, 1992.

Other Specialty Managed Care Arrangements

The costs of long-term, chronic care have forced many specialty health care providers to develop managed care programs and contracting arrangements with insurers and HMOs. Many of these programs offer alternatives to hospitalization and attempt to provide needed services on a less costly basis. Among those specialty programs rapidly developing managed care contracting arrangements are skilled nursing facilities, subacute care, hospice programs, home health services, and rehabilitation facilities.

Many of these specialty providers organize themselves into entities that can contract with insurers, PPOs, and HMOs. Only a few have contracts to serve one plan exclusively. A variety of reimbursement mechanisms are used in these contracts, ranging from discount fee-for-service payments to some form of capitation.

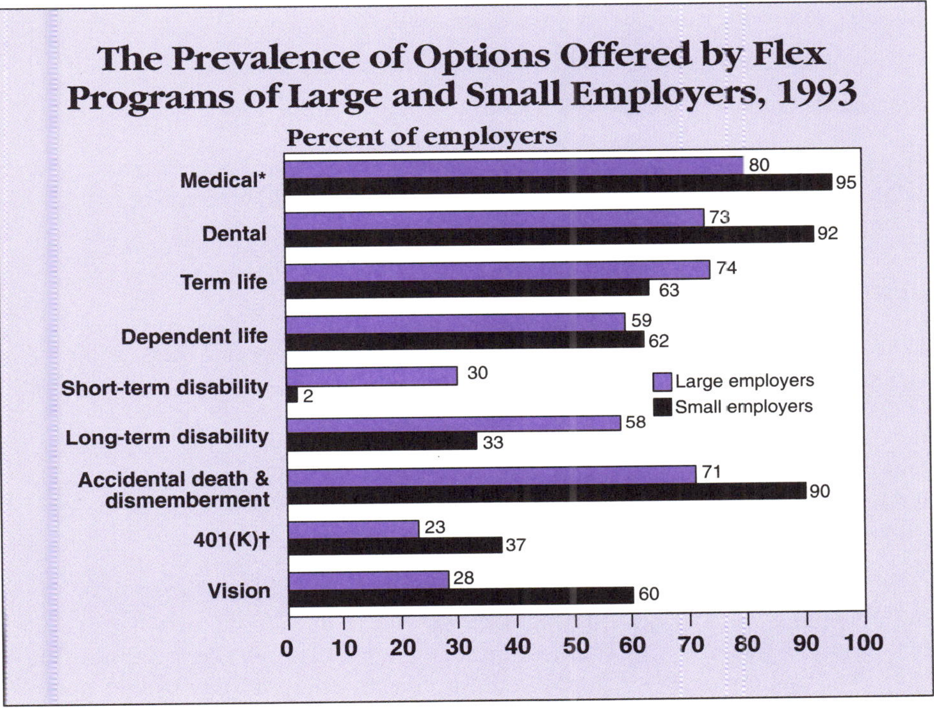

Figure 3.3

*Other than HMOs.

+Within Flex programs.

SOURCE: Foster Higgins National Survey of Employer-Sponsored Health Plans, 1993.

New specialty provider services are being developed, and there is much variability among quality and cost-effectiveness of programs that currently exist. Demands by employers and other payers are forcing these specialty providers to develop standardized programs and measures of service in order to remain viable in a competitive marketplace.

Managed Indemnity

Traditional fee-for-service insurance plans have adopted several managed care techniques for cost containment that they offer to employers/purchasers of insurance. Most common are:

51

- utilization review, including preadmission certification;

- use of specialty organizations to manage utilization; and

- case management in high-cost chronic or catastrophic cases.

While managed indemnity plans offer the least control of any managed care arrangement, they do provide some options for containing some costs.

Centers of Excellence

Many managed care plans use centers of excellence. These are medical institutions that provide advanced forms of treatment (for example, organ transplants and cancer therapies). They are chosen based on their volume of cases, their outcomes and reputations, their location, and their willingness to negotiate fees. Employers are seeking managed care plans that utilize centers of excellence to meet their employees' needs for specialized care. In some cases, employers contract directly with centers of excellence.

Case management frequently makes use of these centers of excellence, along with hospitals, rehabilitation facilities, home health agencies, and other providers. It allows patients with catastrophic or terminal illness to be freed from the stress and anxiety of seeking care in a piecemeal fashion. Programs that coordinate every aspect of treatment, from diagnosis to recovery, are beneficial to patients, families, and society as a whole. Many plans also provide hospice benefits for palliative care to terminally ill patients. The case management services offered by managed care provide consumers with the information necessary to make informed choices. Such information and support are of considerable value to families in times of crisis.

■ Factors That Affect Managed Care

Managed care arrangements are continually evolving, because of a changing economic, technological, and social environment. The factors in this environment and their interplay are important to understand in order to grasp the concept of managed care. The most important of these environmental factors are found in Figure 3.4.

The remainder of this curriculum examines these environmental issues and their impact on the current practice and continuing development of managed care.

Factors that Impact on Managed Care

Environmental Factors	Examples
Stakeholders (Those with a stake in cost and quality of service)	Patients and families Payers (employers, insurers, government) Regulators Health care professionals Health care facilities
Expectations	Satisfaction with service Appropriateness of care Access to care Cost-effectiveness Credentialing and training
Knowledge Base	Development of quality indicators Development of practice guidelines Development of outcome measures Development of common databases Development of management information systems

Figure 3.4

■ Summary

Managed care arrangements are constantly evolving, but currently include various types of HMO, PPO, and POS plans. As managed care arrangements have evolved, areas such as behavioral health, prescription drugs, and dental services often have been carved out and included under single-service or limited-service managed care plans.

The development of managed care arrangements is continually affected by a variety of environmental forces that make demands on the health care system for cost-effective, quality services.

■ Key Terms

Access	Capital costs	Claims
Ambulatory care	Capitation	Closed panel
Annual benefit cap	Carve-outs	Coinsurance
Behavioral health programs	Case management	Copayments
Benefits	Centers of excellence	Cost basis
Bulk purchasing	Chronic care	Credentialing
		Deductibles

Dental specialty
programs
Discounted fee-for-
service basis
Drug utilization
review
Employee Assistance
Program (EAP)
Environmental factors
Exclusive Provider
Organization (EPO)
Fee-for-service
Financial risk
Fixed premium
Formulary
Freestanding plan
Gatekeeper
Generic drug
Group model
Group practices
Guidelines
Health Maintenance
Organization (HMO)
Home health services
Hospice
Incentive payments
Individual Practice
Association (IPA)
Insurer
Liability insurance

Limited-service models
Managed care
Managed indemnity
Management Services
Organization (MSO)
Mental health
management
Multiple provider
arrangement
Multispecialty group
Network
Network or mixed
model
Non-network provider
Open panel
Out-of-network care
Partial hospitalization
Peer review committee
Pharmaceutical
services
Pharmacy networks
Physician-Hospital
Organization (PHO)
Point-of-Service (POS)
Plan
Practice patterns
Preadmission
certification
Preferred Provider
Organization (PPO)

Prescription drugs
specialty programs
Primary care physician
Professional review
Protocols
Qualified claims
Quality assurance
Rehabilitation facilities
Self-referral
Single-service HMOs and
PPOs
Skilled nursing facilities
Specialty HMOs
Staff model
Stakeholders
Stop-loss
Subacute care
Supplementary coverage
Therapeutic equivalent
Third-party administrator
Traditional indemnity
insurance
Unbundled
Withhold arrangements
Usual, customary, and
reasonable fees
Utilization management
Utilization review

Chapter 4

COST CONTROL TECHNIQUES

55 *Introduction*

55 *Controlling Costs Through Reimbursement*

59 *Hospital and Physician Hospital Arrangements Compensation*

63 *Controlling Costs Through Contracting and Provider Selection*

67 *The Gatekeeper Role in Controlling Costs*

67 *Utilization Review in Controlling Costs*

71 *Summary*

72 *Key Terms*

■ Introduction

The growth and development of managed care arrangements have created a new environment for various health care system stakeholders. In particular, managed care organizations, providers, consumers, and payers (employers, individuals, and the government) are affected by, and have an effect on, the development of managed care. Most important for the development of effective managed care programs is the interplay between managed care organizations and stakeholders in an attempt to control behavior. This chapter examines the major controls over cost and utilization that are used in managed care.

■ Controlling Costs Through Reimbursement

Provider compensation is an important tool to control costs in managed care plans. Compensation encompasses elements of risk sharing and incentives that may ultimately have an effect on how providers behave. Certainly, risk-sharing arrangements and salaries based on utilization and productivity are an attempt to make providers more conscious of cost. There are several types of compensation arrangements used in managed care plans.

Payment to Primary Care Physicians in Closed Panels

Primary care physician (PCPs) play key roles in managed care. They are the individuals who actually deliver and manage health care and are central to controlling cost and utilization. The PCP provides basic care to the enrollee, initiates referrals to specialists, and provides follow-up care. Reimbursement to PCPs for services takes many forms. The principal types of reimbursement are salary, capitation, capitation with carve-outs, and fee-for-service.

Salary

Frequently, the PCP has a financial stake in the success of the managed care plan. Staff-model HMOs almost always pay physicians on a salaried basis. Often, quality, utilization, and profit goals affect this salaried compensation. Physicians who have risk-bearing arrangements with managed care plans stand to gain or lose income based on their own performance and the performance of other physicians and the plan as a whole. Because the performance of PCPs has a direct bearing on the financial health of the managed care plan, their performance is the target of incentives and risk arrangements. Though salaried physicians may not have income parity with their fee-for-service colleagues, there are other benefits of a salaried arrangement. For example, malpractice insurance, health and life insurance, and pensions are important benefits that are not covered for physicians in private practice, but can be a part of the salaried compensation package.

Sometimes a portion of the physician's salary, typically 20 percent, is withheld until the performance of the health plan is examined at year's end. If the PCPs have been efficient and the financial goals of the organization have been met, the withhold portion is returned to the PCPs. If there are cost overruns, the withhold amount will not go to the PCP, but will be used to offset any financial losses of the managed care plan. In many situations, the withhold percentage can be increased during the year if referral or hospitalization costs are above target. In many instances, a bonus is paid in addition to salary, if utilization is less than expected.

Capitation

Another common approach, particularly for group-model HMOs, is to pay PCPs a capitated amount for performing routine care. To determine the appropriate amount of capitation, PCP services must be carefully defined in order to estimate the total cost for primary care. This determination also may include adjustment for higher-cost patients or categories of patients. The two most frequent adjustments made to capitation are for age and gender.

The PCP is paid the same amount of money each month for each member (e.g., $25 per member per month [PMPM]), regardless of the number of visits or the cost of services. Many HMOs also make a portion of the capitation payment dependent on the number of referrals to specialty care and the number and length of hospital admissions. For example, if the PMPM is $25, $5 per month is set aside and paid to the PCP if targets for referrals to specialty care are met.

Referral Pools

Other reimbursement arrangements establish a capitation pool for referrals or hospital and nursing home services. For example, the PCP is paid $15 PMPM, but another $15 PMPM is set aside for referrals and $20 PMPM is set aside for institutional care. This capitated pool eliminates some risk to the PCP, and the PCP may share in what is left in the pool at the end of the year if utilization targets for these types of services are met. Capitation is a method for controlling utilization by creating incentives to deliver the most cost-effective care by balancing utilization (withholding needed services could increase the need for more costly services later, and providing unnecessary services also adds to cost).

Carve-Outs

Some capitated programs allow certain services that are not included in the basic PCP capitation to be carved out. Carve-outs are often paid for on a predetermined fee-for-service basis and are aimed at assuring that enrollees get certain preventive or maintenance services as a part of their relationship with the HMO. Such services as immunizations, physicals, basic laboratory screening tests and mammography are often carved out of the basic services for which the PCP receives a capitated payment. This approach seeks to enhance the quality of care the enrollee receives by encouraging the PCP to provide such services. The encouragement is the fee-for-service payment.

Fee-for-Service

The fee-for-service managed care arrangement, unlike traditional fee-for-service payments, builds in cost controls through negotiated fees and "global" fees.

Negotiated fees. The negotiated fee is one in which the managed care plan and the provider mutually agree on a set fee for each service. This negotiated rate is usually based on services defined by the Current Procedural Terminology (CPT) codes, generally at a discount from what the provider would usually charge. Because the PCP cannot charge more than this fee, it becomes an incentive for the PCP to provide services in the most efficient manner possible.

Global fees. Global fees are a set negotiated fee that is all inclusive (one fee is paid for the entire range of services provided for a specific episode or episodes of care). For example, a global fee for prenatal care includes laboratory work, other diagnostic tests, and office visits related to pregnancy.

The global fee is actually a budgeted amount the provider receives for a range of services. By following this "budget," the provider is stimulated to produce services that are more cost-effective. In addition, many times global fees are tied to some type of performance measures or targets and take on some features of capitation. If the global fee for a particular service is set at $15, good performance may mean that the PCP did not have to use all of the $15 and, instead, gets to keep the excess. Global fees offer incentives for more cost-effective primary care services in a fee-for-service system.

Specialty Services Reimbursement

The range of specialty services and providers includes specialty physicians (e.g., cardiologists, neurologists, surgeons) and other types of health care professionals such as physical therapists, rehabilitation specialists, psychologists, and social workers. Though specialty providers may, at times, deliver primary care services, most often they deliver services of a specialized nature, outside the general parameters of primary care.

Managed care enrollees have access to specialists in a variety of ways. The more loosely managed, less restrictive plans, such as simple discount PPOs, allow access to physician specialists on demand. These so-called "self-referral" decisions are made by the managed care enrollee and can include the use of providers both in and out of the network. Enrollees choosing network providers have lower out-of-pocket expenses in the form of copayments and coinsurance than those who choose non-network providers.

In the more tightly managed setting, specialty services can only be used if the PCP refers the enrollee to a specialty physician or other specialty service. To obtain specialty care, an enrollee must get approval from the plan before seeing a specialist. The enrollee either calls the plan or talks with the PCP to get approval. In those managed care organizations that do not require enrollees to select a specific physician as their designated PCP, specialist referrals can be made by any PCP in the network or group. In some cases, a medical group may assume full risk for the cost of care through the capitation payment. In this instance, the medical group typically takes greater responsibility for controlling referrals and managing care. However, full-risk capitation is far less common than the mandatory PCP referral to a specialist for specialty care.

A number of multispecialty group practice physicians and some specialists in IPA-HMOs are capitated like PCPs. However, by far the most common method of reimbursement for specialists is discounted fee-for-service with a withhold arrangement. In this arrangement, specialty providers assume less financial risk than primary care physicians. Frequently, a negotiated fee or global fee is used in this fee-for-service arrangement in order to have as much control over costs as possible.

Use of the Resource-Based Relative Value Scale

Resource-Based Relative Value Scale (RBRVS) payments may be the method used to reimburse specialists. The RBRVS was developed by the Health Care Financing Administration (HCFA) of the federal government. The objective of RBRVS was to distribute physician payments in such a way as to encourage the use of primary care services. In the RBRVS, the amount of resources devoted to produce a health care service serves as the basis for the fee that is paid. The RBRVS method is a form of fee-for-service reimbursement. Though it is a more scientific and objective approach to fee schedules than some developed by traditional insurance, it does have some of the same disadvantages of other fee schedules. It must be complemented by incentives for controlling utilization if it is to contribute to the efficient management of care. The managed care arrangement sets reimbursement for specialists and consultants at an agreed-upon RBRVS rate. Then, that rate is discounted. An advantage of this type of fee schedule is that the contracting organization knows exactly what the charges for a given service will be.

■ Hospital and Physician Hospital Arrangements Compensation

Physician Hospital Organizations (PHOs) assume financial risk through such arrangements as the use of global fees for hospital and medical services. Both physicians and hospitals share in the financial risks of PHO contracts with managed care organizations. PHOs gain economies of scale and efficiency and spread their risk by pooling their contracting activities with other providers. In some cases, PHOs contract directly with employers to provide hospital (and in some cases physician) services to employees. In other cases, hospitals contract directly with managed care organizations and insurers to deliver hospital services.

Hospital and PHO providers may be reimbursed in a variety of ways. (Figure 4.1)

Fee-for-Service

Fee-for-service reimbursement, the least controllable method of payment, encourages providers to deliver more services. Many managed care organizations

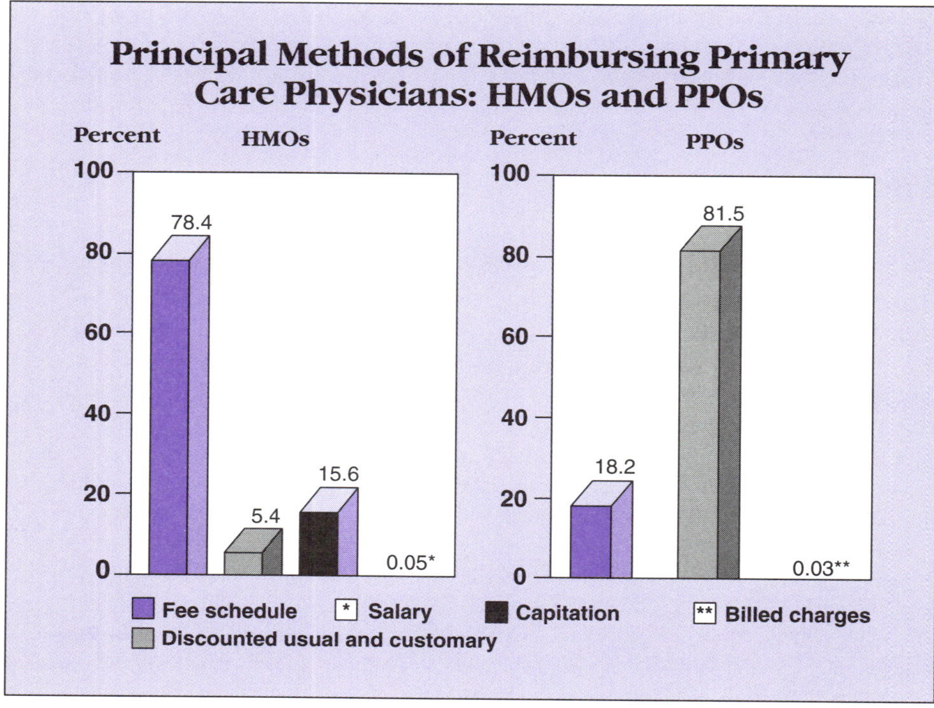

Figure 4.1

SOURCE: HIAA Managed Care Survey, 1990.

negotiate discounted fees with hospitals and PHOs under this reimbursement method. A negotiated discount reduces cost in the short term but does not prevent providers from raising fees or discourage them from providing unnecessary services. To add some degree of cost control, many payment systems make use of the fee-for-service with withhold arrangement. In this type of arrangement, a percentage of the fee-for-service is withheld, as in PCP arrangements, and is released according to performance.

Capitation

Another form of reimbursement is the capitation payment. In this type of risk arrangement (called a risk arrangement because the providers run the risk that the cost of services they provide will exceed the capitation payment), the PHO provider receives a single payment per member, per month (PMPM) to cover the costs of all services provided by the PHO. The PHO has the incentive to provide care efficiently because it is paid only the capitated amount. The PHO is, in effect, on a budget.

The use of capitation for hospitals and PHOs can be more difficult than with the PCP, because the hospital must manage the entire range of services that make up the care. Effective hospital capitation contracts require effective collaboration between physicians and hospitals, because it is the physician who decides what services are to be delivered and it is the hospital that must provide them efficiently.

Case Rates

Hospital and PHOs may also be reimbursed by a managed care organization with which they have a contract on a case-rate basis. Similar to the global fee described earlier, this is a negotiated fixed rate for specific courses of treatment, such as coronary artery bypass grafting. As with the global fee, the case rate can be adjusted to account for those situations requiring more intensive (and more costly) services than usual.

Per Diem

Per diems are fixed rates of payment per day for services rendered. Frequently, managed care organizations specify what services are included in the per diem rate. They are usually paid to hospitals and other institutions for inpatient care and may be limited to a maximum length of hospital stay for a specific diagnosis. Per diem rates can vary substantially, depending on the intensity of services provided. For example, per diem rates for ICU care are much higher than per diem rates for psychiatric inpatient stays.

Diagnosis-Related Groups

The diagnosis-related group (DRG) prospective payment plan is a flat fee for all inpatient services related to a diagnosis and a single episode of care. DRGs came into widespread use after becoming the method of hospital reimbursement for Medicare services in 1983. Because the DRG is considered payment in full for all services delivered during a single episode of care, hospitals and other providers who accept the DRG method of reimbursement from managed care organizations are assuming considerable risk. (Figure 4.2)

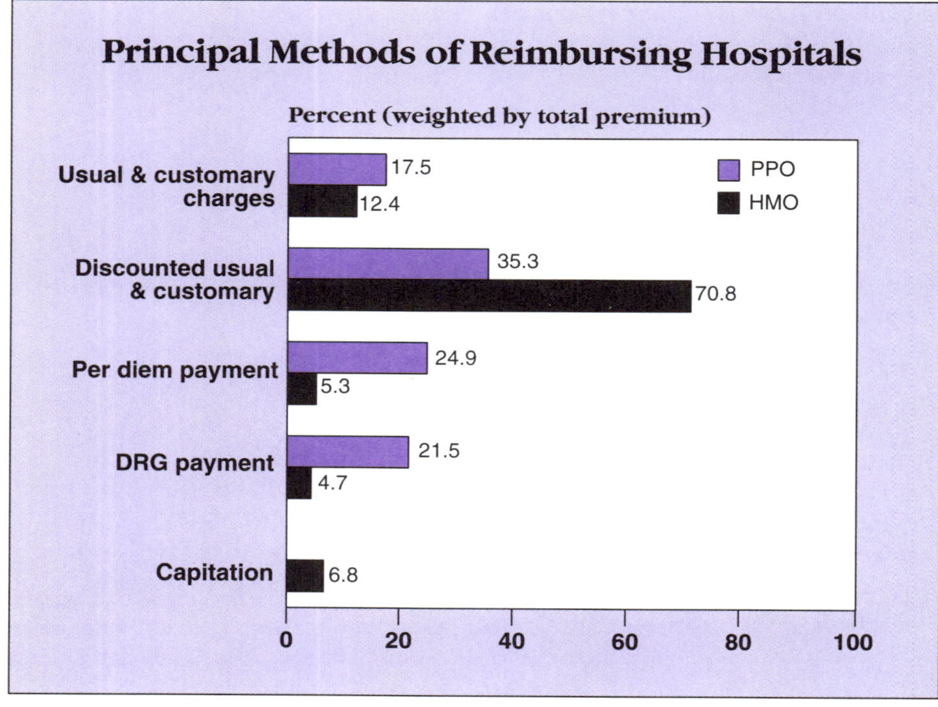

Figure 4.2

SOURCE: HIAA Managed Care Survey, 1990.

Fee Schedules

Fee schedules are comprehensive lists of fees for specific services. They are usually applied as the upper limit of what a payer is willing to pay for specific services. They are intended to increase patient awareness of and responsibility for costs as well as establish a finite limit on what will be paid for any given service. Fee schedules have considerable disadvantages. While fee schedules limit payers' and purchasers' costs, they are often adjusted annually based on a medical inflation index or other predetermined amounts. They also may cause providers to "balance bill," that is, bill the patient for the remainder of the fee, thus shifting costs from the payer to the patient. Another disadvantage is that fee schedules do not address overutilization or underutilization on the part of the provider.

Discounted RBRVS Rates

Discounted RBRVS rates are used with PHOs in a fashion similar to that of specialty care, as described earlier. RBRVS fees for defined services are agreed upon at the outset.

Controlling Costs Through Contracting and Provider Selection

A significant area of control for any managed care organization lies in the area of selection of participating providers. Several methods can be employed to select providers who operate in a cost-effective manner and who work in concert with the goals of the managed care organization. Selecting an efficient, cost-effective provider network is crucial to cost containment and the marketability of managed care.

Optimum network size and selection require the ability to balance marketing and management. In developing and maintaining networks of providers, managed care organizations analyze the market they intend to serve. They must have the ability to attract the right number of effective providers by:

- offering a volume of patients;

- effectively administering provider contracts; and

- enlisting highly qualified and cost-conscious providers to help supervise the network's medical and financial performance.

The managed care contractor seeks to balance an adequate distribution of specialty providers with an adequate number of primary caregivers. In addition, the contractor also seeks to determine the volume and cost of services of potential providers by assessing their previous performances as a measure of how they may perform in the future. One method of assessing performance is the use of physician profiles to retrospectively evaluate a provider's performance.

Recent developments in the physician selection process include the use of profiles that compare physicians' performances to those of their peers, community, or specialty norms of practice to determine a rating.

Hospitals in a managed care network are selected according to the range of services they provide, mortality and morbidity rates for certain illness and disease categories, success at treating patients within cost limits, and reputation in the

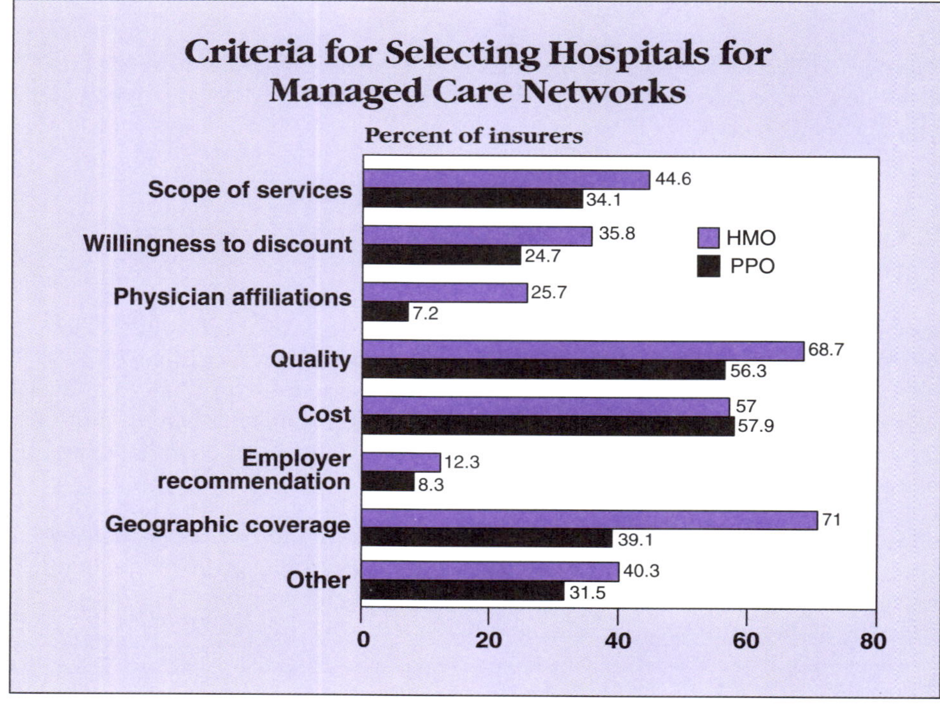

Figure 4.3

SOURCE: HIAA Managed Care Survey, 1990.

community. The correct ratio between cost and the provision of service is crucial to each hospital. (Figures 4.3 and 4.4)

Credentialing

Before hiring or contracting with any providers, an examination of professional credentials is imperative. Professional credentials provide the managed care organization with knowledge of the quality and acceptability of physician practice. Credentials are developed as a result of physicians taking appropriate medical licensing examinations to allow them to practice medicine. Successful completion of an examination allows a physician to be licensed by a medical examination board.

Unlike the traditional indemnity insurer who does not examine the credentials of physicians, managed care organizations are generally very careful to deter-

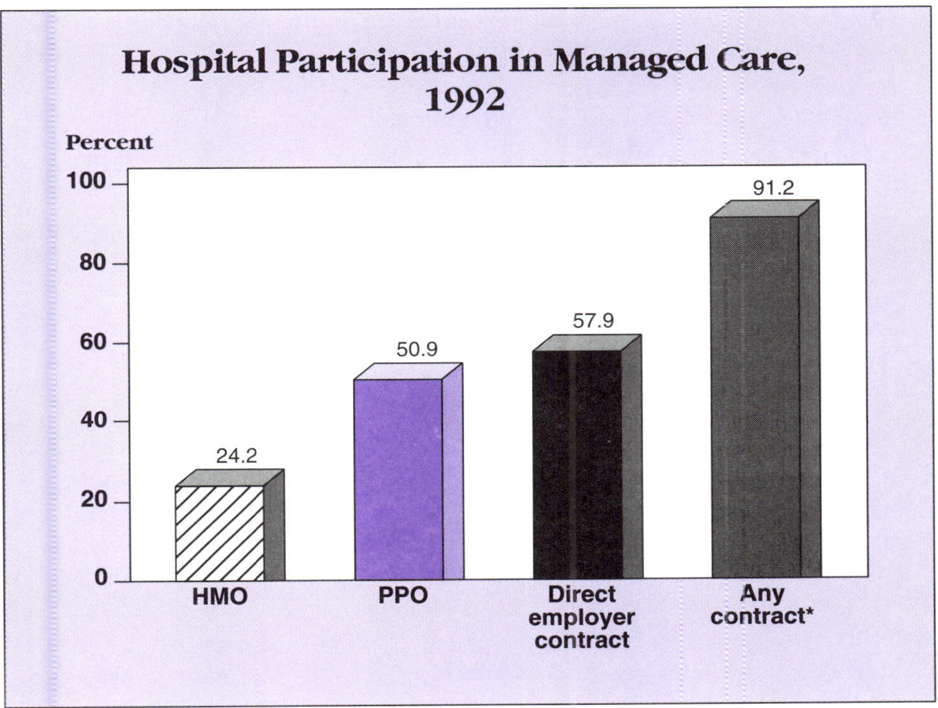

Figure 4.4

*Also includes types of other networks, utilization review, and case management contracts.

SOURCE: State of the Art of Managed Care 1993–1994: A Special Research Report by the Healthcare Provider Network Section of the Society of Healthcare Planning and Marketing, American Hospital Association, 1993.

mine if a person they are considering for hire or contract is actually certified to perform the services desired. This is important for many reasons, including the need to be certain that the managed care organization has a cost-effective balance of PCPs and specialists.

Physician Profiling

A physician or physician group profile is developed to determine the cost-effectiveness of practice. This may include:

- comparison with other physicians or providers of numbers and types of referrals to specialists;

- comparison with other physicians or providers in the use of ancillary services, such as x-rays and laboratory tests;

- comparison with other physicians or providers for numbers of visits or length of hospital stay required to treat certain conditions;

- comparison with other physicians or providers of actual claims cost per patient; and

- medical record review, where a sample of a provider's records are confidentially reviewed by peers to determine effectiveness of treatment and the adequacy of documentation.

Physician profiles are developed from a variety of data sources including:

- claim forms in a fee-for-service environment, or physician-completed patient encounter forms in a capitation environment;

- utilization reviews, or assessment of appropriate use of medical services such as the amount of laboratory testing done and the tendency to refer to specialists;

- analysis of the panel of patients who receive services, including analysis of the percentage of various diseases treated, the age distribution of patients, and the proportion of inpatients to outpatients;

- health status surveys completed by patients, to determine any improvement in health status following medical intervention (outcomes measurement); and

- enrollee satisfaction surveys demonstrating perceptions of quality of services.

Malpractice History

The process of selecting providers also should include an examination of the provider's malpractice history. While malpractice suits are not necessarily an indication of quality of practice, a careful examination of such records is wise.

Malpractice suits and other related reference checks can be obtained through the National Practitioner Data Bank that was developed as a result of the Health Care Quality Improvement Act of 1986. The Act requires health care provider organizations and insurers to report malpractice cases that have been settled or lost. Because this database is relatively small at this time, other methods of checking on malpractice suits include court documents, review journals of court cases, and state medical boards.

Clear Expectations

The managed care organization that wants to select cost-effective providers must make clear its expectations and requirements. Many times, this clarity helps ensure a supply of providers that is practicing or willing to practice medicine in a manner consistent with the organizational goals of the managed care plan.

■ The Gatekeeper Role in Controlling Costs

Another control for cost and utilization in many managed care organizations is the gatekeeper role. A gatekeeper is most often the key to seeking care in a Health Maintenance Organization (HMO) or Exclusive Provider Organization (EPO). The gatekeeper, generally a PCP, directs, manages, supervises, coordinates, and provides basic care to a managed care enrollee. This means that all nonemergency care can only be provided by, or authorized by, the gatekeeper. While the gatekeeper role is not used as a cost control mechanism in many Preferred Provider Organizations, PPOs frequently have instituted this role for the PCP. Often, the gatekeeper role is the basis for other financial risk arrangements such as capitation and referral pools.

Included in the category of primary care gatekeepers are physicians in general practice, family practice, internal medicine, and pediatrics. Although physicians with other specialties, such as obstetrics and gynecology, may deliver primary care in HMOs, they do not perform all the functions of the primary care physician. Often, even when a health plan requires use of a primary care gatekeeper for nonemergency care, an annual visit to an obstetrician or gynecologist is allowed without a referral from the gatekeeper. This is called a limited self-referral option.

Essentially, the gatekeeper role provides control over cost and utilization. The PCP who functions as a gatekeeper controls and channels utilization of services for the managed care organization.

Not all HMOs require the use of a gatekeeper. In some HMOs, a unit within the HMO itself is responsible for referral management.

■ Utilization Review in Controlling Costs

Utilization review (UR) is another method of ensuring quality of care within parameters of cost containment. Unlike the retrospective claim audits of traditional insurance, UR evaluates appropriateness of health care before it is delivered in order to help eliminate waste and potential risks to the patient. UR techniques are mechanisms that attempt to control costs by examining whether:

- services provided are medically necessary; and

- services are provided at an appropriate level of care.

UR data are derived either directly from the treating providers and practitioners or from the patient's medical record. Such utilization review services are typically provided in two ways:

1. Insurers or managed care plans frequently operate their own utilization review program. The staff that support the program and its policies and procedures are all internal to the insurer's operation. They are either employed directly by or, as in the case of specialist reviewers, are paid consultants of the managed care organization.

2. Another common method is for payers to seek such services from independent utilization review firms. An entire industry has evolved to fill the need for utilization review. An estimated 300–400 independent review firms have thousands of contracts with insurers and employers.

A number of different public and private studies on the cost-effectiveness of utilization review have been conducted. A widely publicized report by the Congressional Budget Office on the effects of utilization review applied to traditionally insured populations suggests that these approaches may be effective, particularly when applied to insured groups with exceptionally high patterns of hospital use.[34]

UR programs are used by every type of managed care organization. Some are more formal than others. The most common components of a UR program are listed below.

Case Management

Case management is used for serious, complicated, and protracted conditions such as prematurity, major trauma, cancer, and AIDS. Case managers (usually nurses) handle each case individually, identifying the most cost-effective treatments for these extremely resource-intensive conditions. The case manager works with physicians and other health professionals as well as patients and family members in planning the care. A catastrophic case that is properly managed maximizes health care benefits for the patient, who might otherwise find access to resources limited by benefit maximums.

A substantial number of employees enrolled in programs with a managed care feature are eligible for large claims case management. (Figure 4.5)

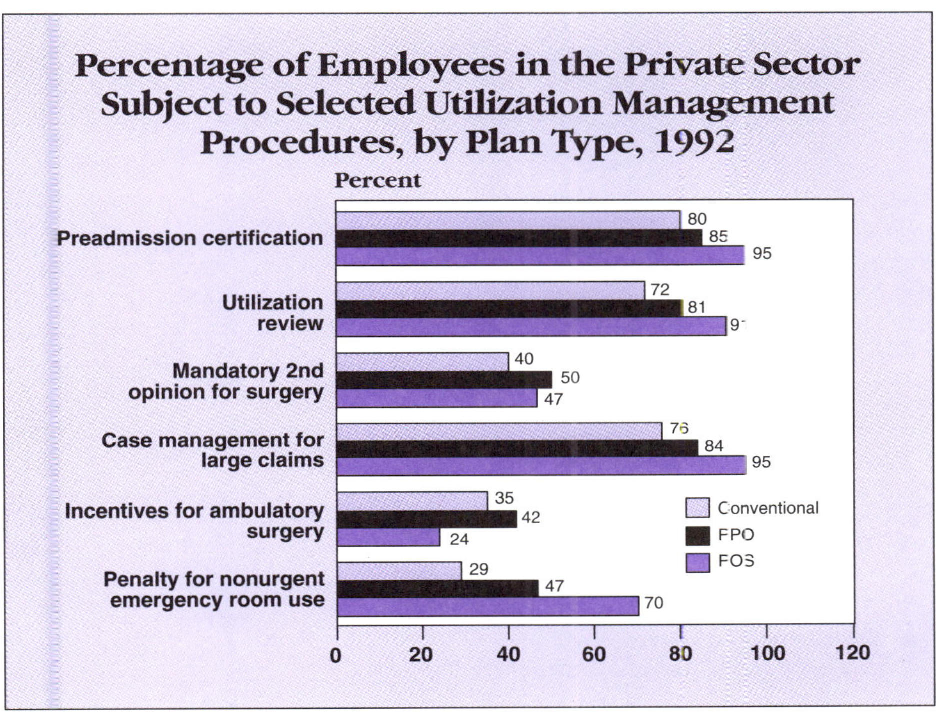

Figure 4.5

SOURCE: HIAA Employer Survey, 1992.

Inpatient Utilization Review

Inpatient utilization review (UR) involves several components which, when combined, make up a significant portion of a utilization management program.

Prospective Reviews

Prospective reviews can take several forms as described below.

Preadmission Certification

Preadmission certification determines, before a patient is admitted to the hospital, the appropriateness of the setting, procedure, or length of stay. The system identifies, whenever possible, outpatient alternatives for care. If a hospital stay

69

is needed, the proposed length of stay and procedure requested are compared with norms to determine appropriateness. Preauthorization determines if a proposed treatment is medically necessary and, if so, authorizes payment for services. If the treatment being proposed is deemed not necessary or appropriate, payment is not authorized.

Usually, registered nurses conduct the initial review of the hospital admission via telephone with the physician who is recommending the hospitalization. Primary care and specialty physicians provide additional clinical expertise during the review process when required. Recent advances in information systems have made computer-assisted decisionmaking and tracking commonplace in the utilization review process. Often, decision protocols are kept on-line; patient specific information may be stored electronically as well.

Outpatient Precertification

One common method of preauthorization is outpatient precertification. Outpatient precertification is most frequently employed to determine the appropriateness of outpatient procedures, such as surgery. It is also used to monitor home health care and the provision of medical equipment in the home, as well as the use of high-risk, high-cost diagnostic evaluations. It is conducted in much the same manner as preadmission certification.

Referral Authorizations

Another common method of preauthorization is referral authorization. Authorizations for referral to specialists and specialized care are made by the gatekeeper PCP or the managed care organization's utilization review program.

Referral authorizations are often made for a single visit. This authorization is a control that forces review after one authorized specialist visit. Claims are not paid for more than one visit.

Concurrent Review

Concurrent review verifies the need for continued hospitalization and determines the appropriateness of treatment rendered in the hospital setting. It is sometimes conducted on-site by a nurse reviewer who examines medical records and interviews the patient's caregivers (and sometimes the patient and patient's family) to determine whether the length of stay and treatment seem appropriate for the condition.

Discharge Planning

Discharge planning determines the need for, and manages the care that a patient may receive upon discharge from the hospital. Discharge planning is generally done by registered nurses in instances where there is a need for continuing care. It is often integrated with concurrent review and case management and helps meet the objective of planning for the most appropriate and cost-effective alternative to inpatient care.

Discharge planning is a method of controlling costs and directing the appropriate services upon discharge from a hospital. Discharge planning should occur as early as possible in a patient's hospital stay. For patients who have not fully recovered or do not require the highly specialized and expensive services of hospital care, discharge planning ensures that the patient receives the most timely, appropriate, safe, and cost-effective discharge.

Retrospective Claims Review

Retrospective claims review examines appropriateness of care that has been delivered in order to determine what costs should be reimbursed. The typical hospital retrospective claim review uses various claim-screen devices, an initial clinical review by nurses, and clinical review by physicians and consultants.

Some typical indicators that may be used to screen claims in order to determine if effective medical care has been provided include readmission for the same diagnosis within 30 days of discharge, or an emergency room visit after discharge from the hospital.

Retrospective utilization review is the evaluation of the necessity and appropriateness of services after they are rendered.

Postpayment Utilization Review

Several postpayment review criteria can serve to determine how well, in retrospect, a physician or physician group is performing.

■ Summary

Providing high-quality health care services that are medically necessary, appropriate for the level of care needed, and cost-effective is the primary concern of managed care organizations. To accomplish this, managed care organizations use certain controls to manage cost-effective care. Among the most common are compensation methods, utilization controls, and selection controls.

By using these controls, it is clear that managed care organizations affect the practice patterns of health care providers. Unlike traditional indemnity insurers, managed care organizations do more than merely pay claims. They attempt to manage the quality, appropriateness, utilization, and cost of care. The impact on the medical profession of managed care is a significant factor in changing the way medicine is practiced in the United States. Efforts to enhance quality, efficiency, and cost-effectiveness are becoming the norm.

■ Key Terms

Appropriateness of care
Authorization reviews
Average length of stay
Balance billing
Capitation
Carve-outs
Case management
Case rates
Claim-screen devices
Coinsurance
Concurrent review
Congressional Budget Office
Contracting
Copayments
Cost-effectiveness of practice
Credentialing
Current Procedural Terminology (CPT)
Defined services
Designated PCP
Diagnosis-related group (DRG)
Discharge planning
Discount
Discounted RBRVS rates
Fee-for-service

Fee schedules
Gatekeeper
Global fees
Health Care Financing Administration (HCFA)
Health Care Quality Improvement Act of 1986
Hospital admissions
Hospital utilization management
IPA-HMOS
Malpractice
Medical necessity
Medical record review
Multispecialty clinics
National Practitioner Data Bank
Negotiated fees
Non-network providers
Norms of practice
Outcome measurement
Out-of-pocket expenses
Outpatient precertification
Overutilization
Per diem

Per member per month (PMPM)
Physician or group profile
Practice profile
Preadmission certification
Preapproval
Preventive services
Primary care
Primary care physician (PCP)
Prospective utilization review
Readmission
Referral
Referral authorizations
Referral pool
Reimbursement system
Resource-Based Relative Value Scale (RBRVS)
Retrospective claims review
Retrospective utilization review
Risk arrangements
Secondary referral controls

Selection controls
Self-referral
Simple discount PPOs
Single-visit
    authorizations
Specialty care

Specialty services
Stakeholders
State medical
    examination boards
Utilization
Utilization management

Utilization review (UR)
Utilization review
    organization
Withhold arrangement

Chapter 5

INDIVIDUALS, EMPLOYERS, AND MANAGED CARE

75 *Introduction*

75 *Individuals and Managed Care*

77 *Changing Consumer Choices*

79 *The Effect of Wellness and Prevention Programs in Controlling Costs*

81 *Consumer Influence on Managed Care*

81 *The Employer and Managed Care*

84 *Employer Influence on Managed Care*

86 *Other Business Arrangements in Managed Care*

88 *Summary*

89 *Key Terms*

■ Introduction

As discussed in Chapters 3 and 4, the impact of managed care on medical providers has been significant. It has made changes in the way medicine is practiced, in the way physicians organize, and in the methods of financial reimbursement. Managed care also has had significant effect on individual consumers of health care as well as on employer groups that insure their workers. This chapter examines the effect of managed care on individuals, employers, employer associations, and unions.

■ Individuals and Managed Care

As with most goods and services, the lower the price, the higher the consumption Since the out-of-pocket price is often well below what it costs to produce the product—in many cases, zero—consumers often purchase an excessive amount of health care. Even if we acknowledge that medical providers, not just consumers, influence consumption decisions, the result is probably similar: when insurers or employers pay the bill rather than consumers, providers and consumers are likely to be less concerned with economizing. In either case, the result is higher than optimum levels of consumption, high medical costs, and inefficient resource allocation.

Cost Sharing as a Control

Until relatively recently, people with insurance acted as if cost was not a factor when consuming health care. Increases in health care costs and the growth of managed care programs have changed this scenario. Before the advent of managed care and flexible benefit plans, the primary vehicle for influencing consumer behavior in traditional indemnity insurance was through cost-sharing features in the benefit design. These benefit design changes sought to give the consumer a financial stake in health care consumption. The most frequently used cost-sharing features were coinsurance and deductibles, which gave consumers a direct financial incentive to obtain care in the most cost-effective setting and to avoid care that was not medically necessary. Coinsurance is the percentage of incurred medical expenses that the patient must pay. A deductible is a specific amount of out-of-pocket expense an individual must pay before being eligible to receive insurance benefits. These methods had some effect on reducing utilization, especially for those services consumers considered frivolous. Unfortunately, they also acted as disincentives to prevention and early intervention, which may have made health care more costly in the long run.

For some time, traditional indemnity insurance has included consumer cost-sharing provisions. Initially, the out-of-pocket expenses associated with these plans were too small to make consumers cost-conscious. Moreover, the effect of the incentives was eroded over time by inflation, rising real income levels, and multiple sources of coverage. Beginning in the late 1960s, and throughout the 70s and 80s, insurers and many employers responded by increasing the level of consumer cost sharing to the point where people were strongly encouraged to weigh carefully the benefits of care against costs before consuming medical services. Today, indemnity benefit plans with deductibles of $1,000 or more and 60/40 coinsurance are fairly common.

Controls for Inappropriate Utilization by Consumers

Cost controls have been built into many indemnity plans as a way of controlling inappropriate use of services. Certain services such as emergency room (ER) services have been sought by individuals even when more cost-efficient and appropriate care is actually needed. The reasons for inappropriate use of services usually are based on availability or lack of direction to the most appropriate provider. Therefore, these services and others have become the subject of cost controls.

People often visit emergency rooms for nonemergency reasons because the ER is open 24 hours a day and because their benefit plan usually does not encourage development of a close relationship with a physician who can provide continuous care, which would eliminate the need for many ER visits. (This is a key reason primary care physicians are required in most HMO-type plans). In an attempt to curb inappropriate use of emergency room services, indemnity benefit plans often include a significant financial barrier that forces the insured to be aware of the cost constraints associated with emergency room utilization. For example, a substantial deductible may be imposed for ER services, requiring the insured to pay the first $200 out-of-pocket before insurance payment occurs.

The Effect of Controls on Utilization

Utilization of ancillary services also is controlled in many indemnity plans. Imposing more substantial cost sharing on ambulatory services gives consumers reason to pause before immediately going to the doctor with minor problems. This is likely to reduce costs in several ways: eliminating the cost of the initial visit and, perhaps more important, avoiding tests and other diagnostic and therapeutic procedures that the provider is likely to order during the visit.

Indemnity controls for hospital care.   Increasing consumer cost sharing for outpatient services must be matched with a corresponding increase in consumers' out-of-pocket costs for inpatient care. When inpatient services are more generously covered than outpatient services, people are hospitalized, often unnecessarily, and usually at higher expense. To prevent unnecessary, expensive hospitalizations, many indemnity plans routinely include prospective utilization review for nonemergency inpatient stays. By coupling the utilization review with appropriate cost sharing, consumers are encouraged to be cost-conscious in making choices to use either inpatient or outpatient services.

■ Changing Consumer Choices

With the growth of managed care and multiple health plan offerings (choice of fee-for-service, PPOs, HMOs, or POS plans), most individuals now face multiple choices at two key decision points.

Choosing a Health Plan

The first choice occurs when the consumer/employee chooses a health plan. Ideally, he or she has a financial incentive to choose the most cost-effective of the options offered. Proper incentives require the employer to pay for less than 100 percent of the premium and employees to pay for the difference between the least expensive plan and other plans. Often, the least expensive plan is a managed care plan that offers the employee a limited choice of providers. Therefore, employees often must choose between a limited choice of providers and higher premiums. In addition, many employees are given a choice of several plan designs, with different benefits and varying degrees of cost sharing. These choices create an additional trade-off between premium contribution and cost sharing.

Out-of-Pocket Expenses

The second critical decision point occurs each time the consumer obtains care. At that point, financial incentives can directly influence the choice to use or not to use services or the choice among various alternative forms of service. For example, individuals enrolled in managed care plans that permit care to be obtained out-of-network generally receive richer benefits when they use network providers and have their care coordinated by a primary care physician whom they select. For most traditional indemnity plans and POS plans, the individual's choices are also greatly influenced by the out-of-pocket costs they incur each time they receive services.

Whether as a single "stand-alone" choice or part of a package of fee-for-service and managed care, the managed care plans contain incentives that influence individual medical care choices and are aimed at achieving greater cost-effectiveness. In some instances, individuals are attracted by richer or more comprehensive benefits. These benefits compensate for the decrease in provider choice in the plans that are more restrictive. In other cases, the difference in degree of cost sharing required among plans or plan levels (e.g., network vs. out-of-network), influences the individual's choice of plan option or type of provider used.

The Effect of Plan Design on Cost Control

Managed care plans have generally placed greater responsibility for cost saving on providers than traditional indemnity plans. Individuals are strongly encouraged, through the plan design, to use network providers. HMOs, for example, typically give network providers strong financial incentives to practice cost-effective medicine while requiring enrollees to use network providers.

HMO plan design typically lets enrollees use non-network providers only in true medical emergencies. Otherwise, they must directly bear the costs for services obtained outside the provider network. In other managed care plans, like PPOs, plan design allows patients the option of selecting non-network providers whenever they choose. In PPOs, the intent is to encourage patients to use network providers. PPO plan design creates incentives to use network providers by requiring patients to bear a significantly higher proportion of the cost when they choose providers outside the plan. A typical PPO plan might cover 100 percent of the cost of care from a network provider but cover only 70 percent of the cost of care from a non-network provider.

POS plans were developed to offer choices not available in a traditional HMO plan design. Like PPOs, the POS plan design allows patients to use providers of their choice whenever they want, for a price. The main difference between POS and PPO plans is that POS plans generally require members to obtain a referral from their primary care physician to receive the richer network benefits. In the past few years, POS plan membership has grown rapidly[35] (accounting for 20 percent of employee enrollments by 1993) because the POS plan design brings the hesitant employer and consumer into managed care through its various incentives coupled with freedom of choice. Other managed care plans are emerging that will combine the freedom of choice that consumers want and cost-sharing elements of successful managed care.

Coordination of Benefits as a Control

If cost sharing is to be an effective deterrent to the consumption of unnecessary care, it is important to preserve the cost-sharing features of a health plan even when there are multiple sources of coverage. One serious problem of the current health insurance system is that many families have more than one source of coverage. Under typical coordination of benefits (COB) provisions, the second plan (or secondary payer) will cover most or all of the consumer co-payments and deductibles that make up the cost-sharing components of the first plan. The result is that the financial incentives for the consumer to economize are eliminated. The care is, in effect, free.

There are various ways to respond to this problem. One approach is to structure COB so that some minimal level of cost sharing is retained regardless of overlapping multiple coverage. A more extreme approach would require changes in the law that allows employers to provide coverage for employees and their dependents only if an employee is the primary family wage earner (or if the primary wage earner has no coverage).

For the present, COB programs for persons with multiple insurance plans have had a negative effect on the incentives that are supposed to be brought about through cost sharing.

■ The Effect of Wellness and Prevention Programs in Controlling Costs

Managed care's coverage of preventive care distinguishes it from traditional indemnity insurance. Despite the common belief that the financial returns on an investment in preventive health are often not realized for decades, it is generally recognized that keeping people healthy is the best way to avoid major health care costs. Because people with no financial barrier to preventive services are more likely to seek early treatment, more serious conditions are prevented from developing to the point of requiring more costly treatment.

Wellness Programs

Most people have the power to influence their health in a positive way through actions that have nothing to do with the health care system. Strong evidence shows that personal behavior is a more accurate determinant of health status than use of medical services.[36] For many people, the choices they make about lifestyle can have more impact on their health than anything the health care system can do for them. Strategies that positively influence people to choose healthy lifestyles deserve support. Recent changes in lifestyle choices among some segments of the population are an indication that educational efforts from many sources can influence people to change in ways that will improve their health. It is hoped that lifestyle changes can help stem the rise in health care costs.

However, one cannot place undue reliance on such programs as a major solution to the health care cost problem. In spite of the great potential to reduce the need for health services by having people adopt healthier lifestyles, it is difficult to induce a significant portion of the population to make the necessary behavioral changes. Nonetheless, insurer promotion of improved lifestyles deserves attention as a way to reduce costs and improve the quality of people's lives.

Preventive Programs as Cost Controls

Consumers should be encouraged to use preventive health services that are truly effective in promoting health. One way to achieve this is to structure cost-sharing mechanisms so that they do not present a barrier to the use of preventive services. It is important to remember that preventive care is a standard benefit in HMO plans, where providers also have stronger incentives to control utilization. Thus, HMOs offer the greatest opportunity to promote health and control costs. The key, however, is to limit this benefit to only those services that have been scientifically demonstrated to be cost-effective, for example, prenatal care, well baby care, and prophylactic dental care.

When medical care is necessary, it is in everyone's best interest to see that consumers know how to use the system most effectively. For many people, the health care system is like a maze or puzzle that is difficult to solve. Insurers can help consumers understand how to get access to the appropriate level of services and, once within the plan, the insurer should provide information on use of preventive services. HMO plans make significant use of several preventive features that are fully covered. These include well baby care, immunizations, and periodic physicals.

■ Consumer Influence on Managed Care

Employees have become more attracted to managed care, primarily because it offers features such as comprehensive benefits at a fixed cost. Because managed care plans want to attract and retain membership, the views of enrollees are regularly solicited in satisfaction surveys and their complaints are heard in grievance processes.

Surveys of managed care enrollees have found a considerable degree of satisfaction with the care received and its cost. Satisfaction tends to increase with the amount of time an individual is enrolled. When offered a choice, 70 percent of respondents to a Gallup poll chose managed care over other options; and they were as satisfied with their health care as were enrollees in traditional indemnity plans.[37] Another survey found that a greater number of respondents (84 percent) were satisfied with their managed care plans than were satisfied with traditional indemnity insurance.[38] It is significant that most of the respondents to both surveys worried more about the possibility of higher premiums than about limitations on their choice of providers.

Increasing use of surveys of managed care members is one development in the evolution of managed care. For the future, managed care organizations can be expected to be more accountable for quality of care and more patient-customer focused.

■ The Employer and Managed Care

Because of the failure of traditional premium-sharing arrangements to address cost inflation problems adequately, many employers have embraced managed care and managed care concepts as a way to control employee benefit costs. The rise in health care costs had a significant effect on employers as the cost of traditional indemnity plans for health care rose steeply in the 1970s and 1980s. As premiums increased at annual rates of up to 50 percent, employers found that traditional arrangements for financing their employees' health care were compromising the profitability, even the viability, of their businesses. A. Foster Higgins, a benefits consulting firm, has estimated that the employer who retains a traditional indemnity plan, even with premium sharing, will be paying over $20,000 in premiums annually per worker by the year 2000, 42 percent more than the projected national average.[39]

Cost containment was not the only issue stimulating employers' interest in managed care. The Health Maintenance Organization Act of 1973 (Chapter 2) stimulated development of HMOs and created HMO-plan features that had greater appeal to employer and employee groups. By 1992, 54 percent of enrollees in employer-sponsored health plans were covered by some type of managed care plan, up from 27 percent in 1987.[40]

Those employers who do not have managed care plans or options available are increasingly including utilization management activities in their conventional plans. Utilization management techniques in managed care (Chapter 4) are an additional aid in lowering health care costs. By 1991, nearly 95 percent of conventional plans used utilization management techniques, compared to only 44 percent in 1987.[41]

Influencing Employee Choices

In the past, many employers provided neither cost-effective health plan options nor any inducement for employees to choose the most cost-effective option offered. In some cases, for instance, employers paid for 100 percent of the premium regardless of the option employees chose. To address this problem, many employers have required employees to pay some portion of the premium, though many premium-sharing arrangements have not provided adequate incentives for employees to choose the most economical benefit structure or the plan with the most tightly managed care.

Over the past ten years, insurers have encouraged employers to elect benefit packages that link stronger cost-sharing limits to the insured's wage or salary level. There are important reasons for trying to link the size of consumers' out-of-pocket payments to their wage or salary levels. The objective is to make the level of out-of-pocket expenses sufficiently high to motivate people to weigh costs and benefits before using services, but not so high as to create major barriers to access for necessary care or to impose undue financial hardship. The particular cost-sharing level that achieves this balance will be different at different income levels: higher for high-income people than for low-income people.

Employer-Employee Premium Sharing Strategies for Cost Control

Premium sharing influences consumer decisions about medical care. It is a strategy that is especially useful when employers design multioption benefit plans for their employees; that is, at the point of enrollment, employees are allowed to choose between two or more benefit plans.

Employer-employee sharing of health insurance premiums is structured so that employees who choose the more expensive plans bear the cost of that choice. This is simply an extension of the economic principle that people should be expected to pay more when they choose to consume goods or services that require more resources to produce.

Consumers must have a financial interest in conserving health resources. But sudden large increases in consumer cost sharing have met with strong resistance from employees. Such increases may also be interpreted as an attempt simply to shift costs away from employers, who can no longer absorb the increases, onto employees. To counter these perceptions, cost sharing is being phased in gradually. In addition, changes should be linked to:

- the insureds' wage or salary levels;
- increases in the cost of medical services (an approach that has the advantage of making consumers very aware of the impact of rising medical costs); and
- the Consumer Price Index.

To preserve the effects of consumer cost sharing over time despite inflation, insurers have advised employers to consider benefit packages that link the magnitude of consumer cost sharing to changes in an appropriate price index, such as the medical care price component of the Consumer Price Index. Such indexing is desirable because the deterrent effect of deductibles and out-of-pocket maximums (but not coinsurance, which is a percentage, not a fixed cost) is eroded as prices and incomes rise. In addition to preserving the deterrent effect of cost sharing, indexing would help make consumers aware of the effects of medical cost escalation in a very direct way, possibly increasing their support for cost containment.

For example, employers often have paid a fixed percentage of the premium cost for all options, but such an approach provides a greater subsidy for purchase of more expensive plans: plans with the greatest freedom of choice, the richest benefits, and/or the least amount of managed care. In addition, the fixed percentage approach has potential for creating adverse selection—for attracting sicker individuals to the least managed plan. Because of the greater subsidy for richer benefits or the opportunity to continue using their own (possibly non-network) specialists, the sickest individuals will increase claims costs in the plan that generally provides the least managed care controls.

Employers are sometimes reluctant to make a commitment to wellness and prevention programs because they are unsure that the benefits will justify the cost of establishing the program. By providing scientifically valid evidence about cost-effectiveness, the insurance industry helps employers make sound judgments regarding the worth of such programs.

■ Employer Influence on Managed Care

Until recently, many employers have been reluctant to embrace managed care wholeheartedly, particularly the HMO model. The main reasons for reluctance to give up the traditional fee-for-service model were concern that employees would be dissatisfied with the perceived lack of choice in HMO plans and concern that early models of managed care such as PPOs did not have effective utilization controls that would actually reduce benefit costs.

This early employer concern had great effect on the development of managed care arrangements and managed care cost control methods.

Purchasers of group and individual insurance can now choose from a variety of benefit plans with a wide range of cost-containment and cost-sharing features. Insurance with multiple plan options from which the employee selects one plan at the point of enrollment are also available to employer groups.

Many large employers have become more active participants in managing their health care dollars, either by setting up their own provider networks or playing a stronger role in managing their benefit plans. More commonly, employers are requesting more detailed data on the utilization of services by their employers and are asking to be "experience-rated" (having their premium rates set on the basis of previous utilization and claim experience) rather than "community-rated" (premium costs set for all employer groups covered by the insurer).

Thus, driven by the need to control costs, employers play a significant role in shaping managed care today. Pressure from employers is causing continual modification of managed care models and products. HMOs have streamlined and diversified their products in response to employer demands. The most striking instance has been the proliferation of POS plans. At the same time, employers are pressing HMOs to provide detailed information and are asking to be experience-rated.

Moreover, employers as a group constitute an extremely influential element in the evolution of health policy because they are the nation's major purchasers of health benefits. Their preferences will continue to influence developments in managed care.

Large Employers

Large employers are helping to design managed care plans. They are requiring acceptable levels of service from the plans that they purchase and are participating in the design of benefit packages. They are scrutinizing not only costs, but also the quality of care and patient satisfaction. They are hiring health care experts to help them evaluate plans by establishing criteria and developing guidelines.

For example, when Xerox Corporation decided to revamp its health benefit program it undertook an exhaustive review of managed care plans. Ultimately, Xerox organized several HMOs into a network and appointed six managed care organizations as network managers who are required to collect utilization and member satisfaction data and to evaluate utilization review and quality management efforts. More than half of Xerox's employees are enrolled in the network.

In other cases, large managed care companies who operate networks on a national level are successfully marketing their managed care products to large employers who operate nationally. These large employers, conducting business in multiple locations throughout the country, are replacing their traditional insurance with a single managed care plan or managed care strategy, such as a POS plan.

Small Employers

While 98 percent of firms with 100 or more employees offer health insurance, only 36 percent of small employers with fewer than 100 employees do.[42] Indeed the smaller the firm, the less likely it is that its employees will enjoy health care benefits. Because small employers tend to employ lower-paid workers and operate under narrower operating margins than do large employers, they are more likely than large employers to find the cost of providing health care prohibitive. Managed care, which restrains costs while it monitors quality, has enabled some small employers to give their workers health care coverage that they would otherwise find unaffordable. At the end of 1991, 8 percent of firms with fewer than 25 employees offered an HMO and 11 percent offered a PPO. Fifteen percent of firms with between 25 and 99 employees offered an HMO and 15 percent offered a PPO.[43]

Small employers have tended to select PPOs because their relatively loose structure makes them attractive to employees unfamiliar with the concept of managed care. Moreover, many of the carriers that had been providing these employers with traditional insurance entered the managed care market with a PPO product, which they then sold to their clients. A growing number of small firms are finding other managed care options, such as EPOs and POS plans, to be appealing.

The flexibility of POS plans has made them increasingly popular with small businesses. Like their larger counterparts, many small employers have replaced their traditional indemnity plans with a POS plan. Small employers are also showing an interest in EPOs, which are more tightly controlled systems than PPOs but require less administration than HMOs. EPOs generally offer lower costs and more control of costs, which appeals to small employers.

■ Other Business Arrangements in Managed Care

In addition to employers, other business arrangements and labor groups also are interested in managed care. These include labor unions and business coalitions and cooperatives.

Labor Unions

From the 1930s onward, labor unions have participated in the creation of HMOs for their members. As health care costs have escalated in recent years and businesses have attempted to implement cost-containment and cost-sharing strategies in the health plans of their employees, tensions between management and labor have risen. Disagreements between management and labor over health benefits have led to bitter strikes, though union leaders seem willing to cooperate with management in containing health care costs through managed care arrangements if the savings are paid to workers in the form of wages or increased job security.

Major issues for union leaders are curbing out-of-pocket employee expenses, counteracting the effects of increased health care costs, and improving health care benefits.[44] The American Federation of Labor-Congress of Industrial Organizations (AFL-CIO) supports managed care as a matter of policy, believing that it has a substantial role to play in controlling costs and monitoring the quality of health care.

Business Coalitions and Cooperative Purchasing Arrangements

Beginning in the late 1970s, business took a leading role in establishing coalitions, which initially served as forums for information sharing, to better understand the factors driving health care cost increases and to identify ways to implement cost-effective benefit plans. Over the last decade, business coalitions began to sponsor cooperative health care purchasing arrangements to contain costs and improve quality.

A 1992 survey by the Dunlop Group of Six reported that, of the 115 coalitions in which business was the primary constituent, 56 were involved in purchasing health care services. In 1994, the National Business Coalition on Health Care, an association of local business coalitions, reported that more than 80 of its organizational members were engaged in cooperative purchasing efforts.

Thus, employer interest in business coalitions has increased with the use of collective purchasing agreements to help reduce health care cost increases. Indeed, small firms have obtained access to managed care by forming coalitions that act as single buying units to pool risk and obtain cost-effective plans.

For example, in Minneapolis, 14 companies of varying sizes formed a coalition and set up a competitive bidding process among several health care providers.[45] This coalition of employers contracted directly with two HMOs and several hospital providers. The competition among bidding providers was based not only on cost, but also on quality, as a growing number of employers are embracing the philosophy that quality is the key to cost-effective medicine. Purchasing arrangements by coalitions are also operational in many other parts of the country, such as Memphis, Nashville, Cleveland, St. Louis, Chicago, Milwaukee, Denver, San Diego, and San Francisco.

Coalitions, some of which originally were formed for other purposes, have found a variety of ways to address health care cost concerns directly. In turn, employers initially concerned about the rising cost of health insurance have targeted coalition efforts to improve quality, as well as lower costs. Among the various strategies being employed are:

- educational efforts directed at employees and families;

- development of uniform, comprehensive information systems;

- development of cost-effective benefit plans;

- use of utilization management programs; and

- use of managed care networks.

Coalitions seek to create market-driven, community-based provider networks through competitive bidding processes. Volume purchasing and competitive bidding have been used effectively in several instances to reduce health care costs, not only for the members of the coalition, but for the community as well.

Coalitions establish or contract with networks of PPOs or HMOs that agree to negotiated payment methods that can include:

- discounted fee schedules of medical services;

- discounted per diem charge for hospitalization; and

- capitation rates or other forms of payment.

Other agreements may restrict or prohibit balance billing by providers, stipulate utilization management programs and requirements, and establish quality measurements and objectives. Establishment of and adherence to requirements for data reporting and other data information services may be included. There is growing interest by coalitions in requiring all providers to use a common and uniform method to report health care data in order to facilitate measurement and comparison of outcomes and quality. (Chapter 7)

In addition to PPOs and HMOs for medical and surgical hospitalization and physicians' services, networks and negotiated arrangements are also often used for:

- treatment of chemical dependency and mental health;

- workers' compensation care (See Chapter 6);

- pharmacy services;

- home health care services; and

- durable medical equipment and other specialized needs.

Utilization and quality management programs may be developed in-house by the coalition or provided through a contract with outside parties. Utilization management program components may include preadmission review, pre-certification of outpatient testing, concurrent and retrospective review, case management of high-cost claims, discharge planning, and hospital bill review. (Chapter 4)

■ Summary

Managed care has had a significant effect on the behavior of individuals and employer groups. It has also been affected by consumer and payer interest in having comprehensive health benefits at reasonable cost. Education and experimentation have been the hallmarks of growth as managed care cost controls have been added to traditional indemnity insurance and as managed care programs have become increasingly popular.

■ Key Terms

Ancillary services
Balance billing
Benefit design
Business coalitions
Capitation rates
Coinsurance
Collective purchasing
   agreements
Community-rated
Competitive bidding
Concurrent and
   retrospective review
Cooperative purchasing
   arrangements
Coordination of benefits
   (COB)
Copayments
Cost sharing

Deductibles
Discharge planning
Discounted fee
   schedules
Discounted per diem
Emergency room
   services
Experience-rated
Fee-for-service
Health maintenance
   organization (HMO)
Hospital bill review
Labor unions
Mental health services
Network providers
Out-of-plan care
Out-of-pocket expenses
Overutilization

Point-of-service (POS)
   plan
Preadmission review
Precertification of
   outpatient testing
Preferred provider
   organization (PPO)
Premium
Provider networks
"Stand-alone" choice
Substance abuse services
Traditional indemnity
   insurance
Utilization
Utilization review
Volume purchasing

Chapter 6

GOVERNMENT INVOLVEMENT IN MANAGED CARE

91 *Introduction*

92 *Medicare*

96 *Other Contracting Methods*

98 *Managed Care and Long-Term Care*

99 *Medicaid*

104 *Military Health Services System*

105 *Federal Employee Health Benefits Program*

106 *Other State Programs*

107 *Workers' Compensation Programs*

112 *Managed Care Alliances*

114 *Summary*

114 *Key Terms*

■ Introduction

The federal government is the largest single purchaser of health services in the United States, paying more than 40 percent of all health care costs through Medicare, Medicaid, and its programs for federal workers, both civilian and military. (Figure 6.1) The increased cost of health care over the past ten years has therefore been a source of serious concern to the federal government, which turned to managed care in the early 1970s.

The Health Maintenance Organization (HMO) Act was a bipartisan initiative, and managed care has been supported by every presidential administration since 1973. But, while the federal government has provided leadership and support through various programs, its commitment has been inconsistent, particularly in the Medicare program.

In addition to Medicare and Medicaid, other government programs have looked to managed care for cost control. The Civilian Health and Medical Program of the Uniformed Services (CHAMPUS), the Department of Defense health programs, and Workers' Compensation are examples of government programs that seek to manage costs more effectively. Many states also have experimented with managed care programs to control rising health care costs for the Medicaid program and to manage workers' compensation costs better.

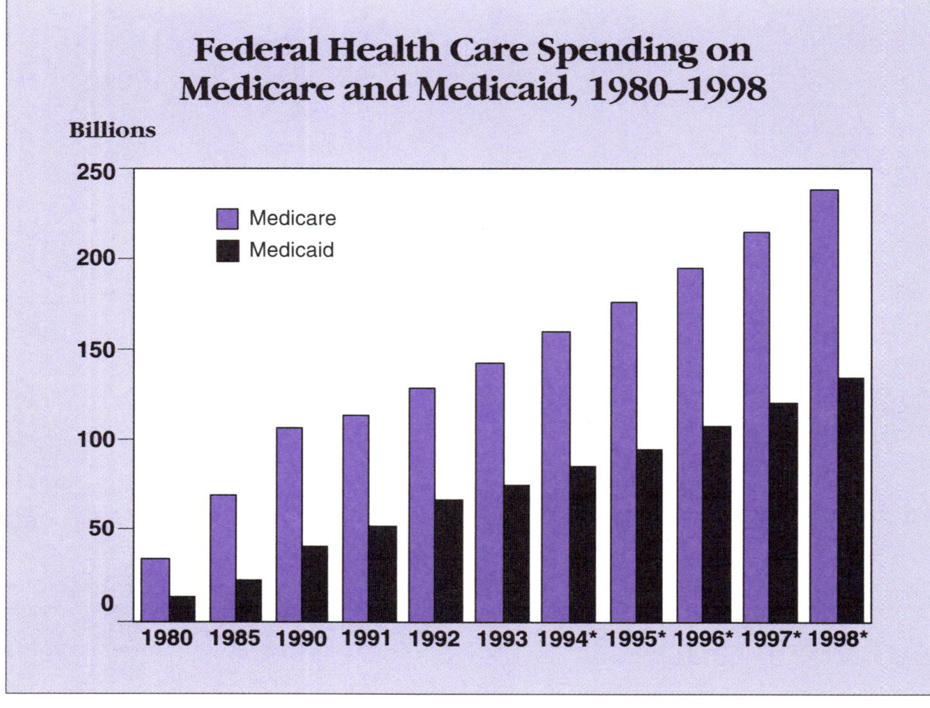

Figure 6.1

*Estimated.

SOURCE: Congressional Budget Office, 1994.

■ Medicare

Medicare is the federally sponsored program paid by employee-beneficiary contributions under the Social Security Act. It provides hospital and supplementary medical benefits to persons 65 years of age and older and to some younger persons who are covered under Social Security benefits. There are two parts to Medicare: Part A pays for hospital services; Part B, which is voluntary, pays a percent of reasonable and customary costs for physician and ancillary services.

Unfortunately, managed care for Medicare enrollees has not achieved the breadth, sophistication, and success of managed care for the private sector. Although these programs have demonstrated success in controlling costs in the private sector, most have failed to enroll enough members to reach the significant cost savings that is within their potential.

Since its early days, Medicare has used fee-for-service payments, in part as a result of pressure from providers. These payments tend to encourage overutilization of health services, as they do in traditional indemnity insurance. As the costs of Medicare have risen, the federal government, which created the legal framework for HMOs in the early 1970s, has turned to those HMOs for help.

Before the passage of the Tax Equity and Fiscal Responsibility Act (TEFRA) of 1982, Medicare coverage through managed care organizations was limited to HMOs that met the criteria for federal qualification under the HMO Act. Because these criteria were difficult to meet and the rate of reimbursement for services under the Medicare contract was often considered inadequate, most HMOs that participated in Medicare did not enter into a prepaid risk contract (a type of capitation program); instead, they were paid on a cost basis, or they billed for individual services, and the cost saving advantages of capitation found in the risk contract were lost. By 1993, 100 HMOs had enrolled only about 5 percent of all Medicare beneficiaries.[46]

HMO Risk Contracts

Medicare's method of funding HMO services for its enrollees is to develop risk contracts with HMOs or competitive medical plans (CMPs). A CMP is "an organization that meets specific eligibility criteria for Medicare risk contracting but is not necessarily an HMO."[47] These eligibility requirements include:

- certification that the HMO/CMP is recognized under state insurance law;

- provision of basic services under Medicare Part A (hospitalization) and Medicare Part B (physicians' services) and various outpatient services;

- HMO/CMP assumption of full financial risk for health care services provided;

- demonstration of adequate financial resources for enrollee protection in the event of insolvency; and

- agreement to accept prospective capitation.

Adjusted Average per Capita Cost

In the risk contract arrangement with HMOs or CMPs, Medicare establishes a prospective capitated payment through use of the Adjusted Average per Capita Cost (AAPCC). The AAPCC is a projected figure based on age, health status, sex, and average health care costs on a county basis. Since managed care is expected to be more cost-efficient than fee-for-service, the government pays a prospective capitated rate that is less than the expected costs per person.

In addition, the Health Care Financing Administration (HCFA) of the U.S. Department of Health and Human Services requires that the AAPCC be compared to the HMO's or CMP's adjusted community rate (ACR), which is a uniform premium rate charged to all enrollees in the plan, based on adjustments for risk factors such as age and sex. If the ACR is less than the AAPCC, the HMO/CMP will either return the difference to the government or lower premiums for Medicare enrollees by the amount of the difference.

In 1980 and 1981, HCFA undertook a series of demonstration projects to test methods of contracting and reimbursement. Eight HMOs, assuming different proportions of risk, contracted to receive capitated payments of 85 to 95 percent of their resident counties' Medicare AAPCC. Between 1982 and 1984 when TEFRA expanded the HMO risk contract demonstrations, 27 HMOs enrolled Medicare beneficiaries. HCFA reimbursed these HMOs at 95 percent of their local AAPCC, which remains the current rate of payment.

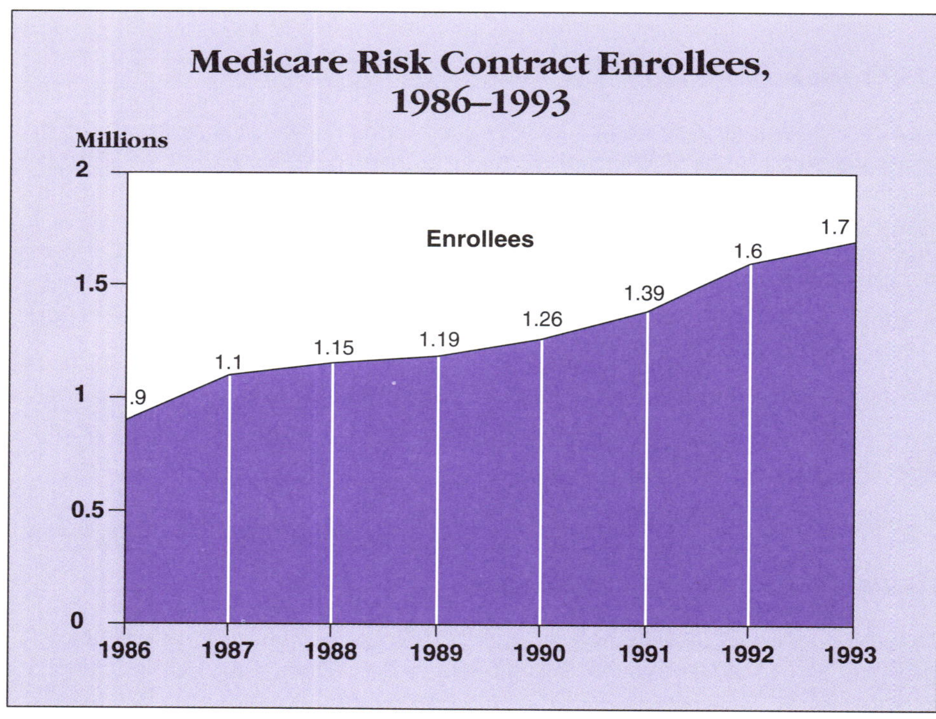

Figure 6.2

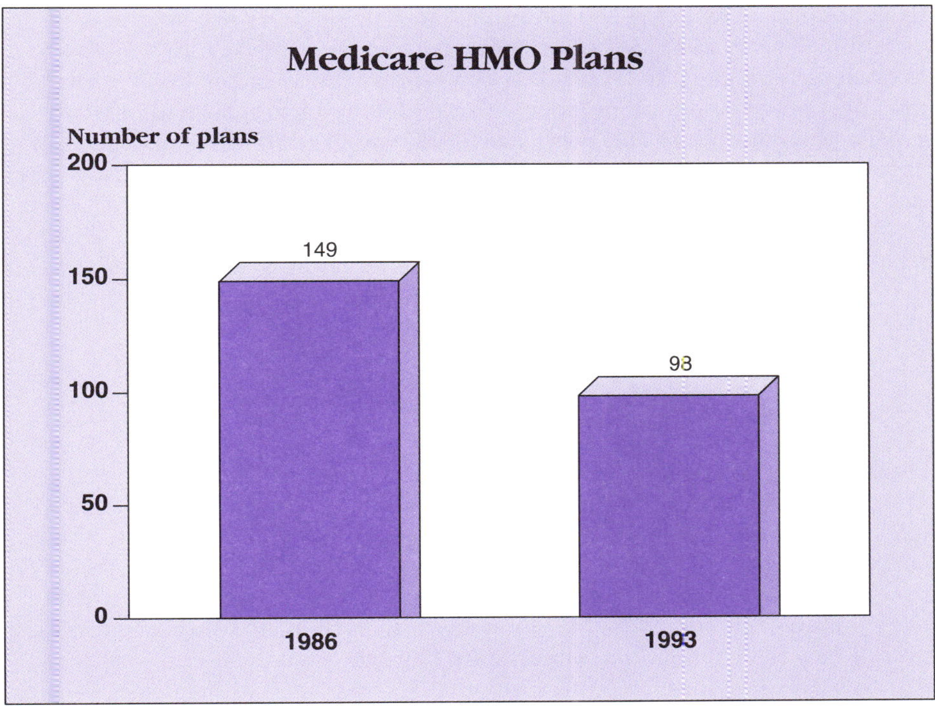

Figure 6.3

SOURCE: Health Care Financing Review, 1993.

Since Medicare risk contracting demonstration projects began in 1980, the number of HMOs participating has widely fluctuated and enrollment growth has been modest. (Figure 6.2) From 1986 to 1993, the number of participating HMOs continued to decline. (Figure 6.3)

TEFRA risk contract programs did not experience a growth similar to that of the general managed care market in the 1980s. Income from the program may be one factor. A survey of HMOs by the Group Health Association of America (GHAA) found that only 53 percent of HMOs reporting Medicare revenues had Medicare operating surpluses in 1989.[48] In 1991, more than half of all TEFRA risk contractors were independent practice association HMOs; the IPAs are the organizations that are less likely than group- and staff-model HMOs to renew their TEFRA contracts. However, over the past few years, there has been some enrollment growth in HMO risk contracts and some renewed interest in Medicare risk contracting on the part of HMOs.

In addition to some dissatisfaction by HMOs with Medicare risk contracts, the government also has shown some concern about their efficacy. In a 1994 General Accounting Office study,[49] it was estimated that such contracts forced the government to pay more money than if enrollees had remained in fee-for-service Medicare plans. This is because those enrollees who choose HMO/CMP Medicare programs are generally younger and healthier retirees. Because of the rich benefit programs of HMOs, these people tend to use more health care services than if they were in traditional fee-for-service, cost-sharing plans. Also, as Medicare beneficiaries age, and experience more illnesses, they tend to drop out of the HMO/CMP programs and join more traditional indemnity plans that allow less controlled use of specialists and services.

Cost Contracting

HMOs undertook cost contracting for Medicare beneficiaries as a alternative to risk contracting. At first, because HMOs did not have adequate systems for tracking costs and billing on a cost reimbursement basis, HMO participation in cost contracting was limited. However, risk contractors, experiencing difficulty because of inadequate AAPCC rates and high utilization of services by the elderly, increasingly turned to cost contracts, which protected them against loss even if they denied them the opportunity to make profits. But cost contracting does not give providers incentives to practice cost-conscious medicine. For this reason, HCFA is critically examining Medicare cost contracts to determine their cost management efficacy.

■ Other Contracting Methods

HCFA is attempting to address some of the problems of risk and cost contracting described above, while at the same time understanding that HMOs/CMPs need to at least break even. Medicare is studying more effective ways to encourage use of HMOs/CMPs in an attempt to gain the cost savings of managed care.

Medicare SELECT

The Medicare SELECT program, a product of the Omnibus Reconciliation Act of 1990 (OBRA-90), has been designed to introduce Medicare beneficiaries to managed care systems through supplemental (MedSup) health insurance. Approximately 70–75 percent of Medicare beneficiaries have MedSup insurance.[50] MedSup supplements Medicare Part B, which does not pay for all nonhospital costs and services. The SELECT plans provide MedSup coverage through PPOs as an incremental way of familiarizing enrollees and providers with utilization management techniques and the use of defined provider networks.

Medicare SELECT demonstrations were authorized in 15 states at the beginning of 1992. Before that date, only one demonstration model, Blue Cross and Blue Shield of Arizona, was operational. The success of these demonstrations will depend upon the extent to which participants can enroll Medicare beneficiaries in existing provider networks, create incentives for enrollees to use network physicians, and arrange discounts with providers in a market already discounted by Medicare reimbursement.

Health Care Prepayment Plans

HCFA allows for a health care prepayment plan (HCPP) for managed care groups that organize, finance, and deliver Medicare Part B services only. HCPPs also may elect to be reimbursed on a "reasonable cost basis."

To qualify for reasonable cost reimbursement, the HCPP must:

- enter into a written contract with HCFA;
- furnish physician services through its employees or under a formal arrangement with medical groups, IPAs, or individual physicians; and
- furnish other covered Part B services through Medicare-qualified providers.

HCFPs allow for more limited and controlled Medicare managed care services to a somewhat reluctant population of older people who are not familiar with managed care arrangements.

Point-of-Service Plans

HCFA is designing a Point-of-Service option, which, like the SELECT program, is specifically intended to introduce Medicare beneficiaries to managed care. The initial HCFA design lacks the structural advantages and incentives of existing POS plans, which may limit its effectiveness. However, the Medicare POS is still under design at the time of this text's publication and will undoubtedly undergo further modification and experimentation.

HMO Group-Only Plans

HCFA is also considering an HMO group-only contract that would enable retiring workers who are already enrolled in employer-sponsored HMO programs to receive Medicare health benefits through their HMOs. Participating HMOs would enroll employer-sponsored groups on a capitated basis, but need not participate in the regular risk contract program. Instead, HMOs would experience-

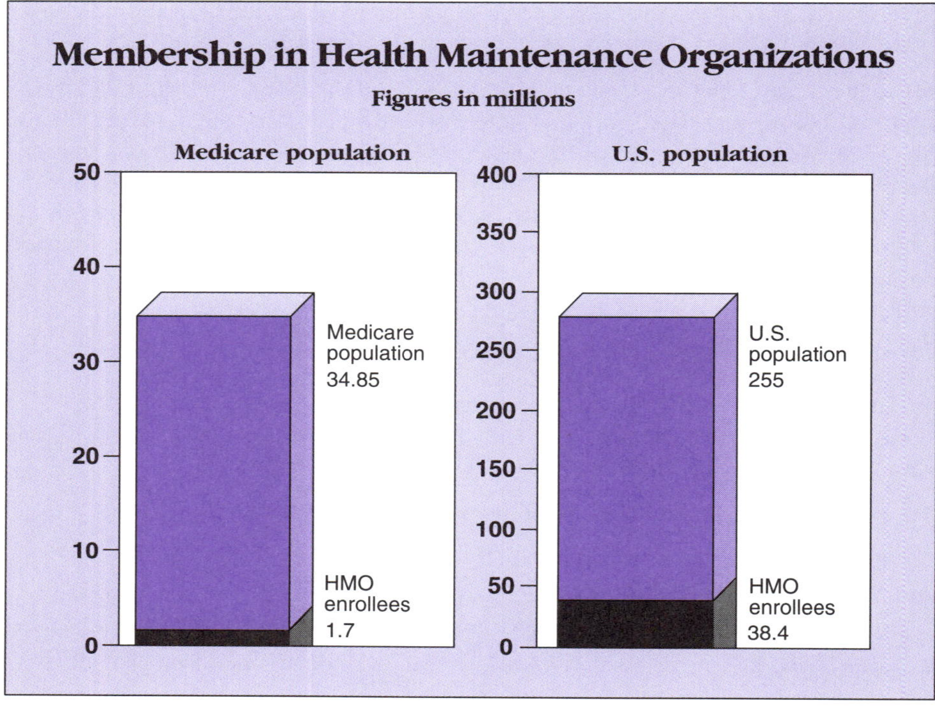

Figure 6.4

SOURCE: Health Care Financing Review, 1993.

rate groups (set premium rates based on previous claims and utilization), and HCFA would use those rates, rather than Medicare AAPCC rates, to determine payment levels. This plan promises to be appealing to retirees, their employers, and their HMOs.

After more than a decade of Medicare risk contracting, only 4.9 percent of those eligible for Medicare receive health care in managed care settings. The enrollment of the Medicare population in managed care is significantly lower than that of the population as a whole. (Figure 6.4)

■ Managed Care and Long-Term Care

Over the next 30 years, the proportion of the population of the United States that is over the age of 65 will grow from 12 percent to 18 percent; fastest growing of all will be the population over the age of 85. This population consumes disproportionate quantities of health care. Today, one-third of spending for health care in the United States is done by and for the elderly, and that proportion will increase.[51] A more complete integration of Medicare with managed care could address the considerable problem of delivering affordable health care to the elderly. Since a significant portion of government financial involvement in health care is related to the elderly, improvement in managing health care for this population would benefit the entire country.

Unfortunately, managing health care for the elderly means managing long-term, chronic care costs. At the present time, Medicare covers very few long-term care needs, such as nursing homes, custodial care, adult day care, or assisted living. Private insurance is a very small source of long-term care protection, covering less than 5 percent of the eligible population.

Some federal experimentation has occurred through funding of managed care demonstration projects. One major demonstration program funded four Social Health Maintenance Organizations (SHMOs) that use managed care principles for the long-term care population. A capitation payment is made for each participant, and case management is emphasized. Enrollees are directed to less expensive, noninstitutional care, and many of the services provided through case management are not regular benefits of Medicare. This experimentation is yielding information on questions such as whether managed care principles can be effective in reducing long-term care costs, and whether use of nontraditional Medicare benefits can provide higher-quality, more satisfying services to aged individuals with chronic care needs for a reasonable cost.

Much work remains for the health insurance and managed care industry in addressing the changing needs of society for long-term, chronic care from the short-term, acute care model of the past.

■ Medicaid

Medicaid is a state-run program (with matching federal funds) for public assistance to persons, regardless of age, whose income and resources are insufficient to pay for health care.

As state and local governments find themselves in financial crisis, they look toward Medicaid, the fastest rising item in state budgets, as a possible place to cut costs. In fact, recent federal mandates requiring expansion of Medicaid benefits to additional populations have actually contributed to the states' fiscal crises. In response, states have lowered benefits and increased eligibility requirements. Medicaid program enrollment reached an estimated 30.1 million in 1992, with program expenditures estimated at $127.2 billion.[52]

For some time, states acted slowly and tentatively in implementing managed care for Medicaid, but that trend is changing. Today state-managed care programs enroll 3.6 million Medicaid recipients, 13 percent of the nation's Medicaid population.[53]

Previous Managed Care Efforts

Before 1981, several provisions of the federal Medicaid statute prevented states from implementing managed care initiatives unless they first undertook formal demonstration projects. In the early 1970s, a few states, notably California, Michigan, and New York, established programs to encourage the voluntary use of prepaid, capitated plans by Medicaid recipients. However, because of unscrupulous marketing practices by some of these plans in California, the federal government imposed further restrictions in 1977.

From 1977 to 1981, states were allowed to enroll Medicaid recipients in prepaid, capitated health plans if they met certain requirements: No more than 50 percent of the plan's enrollees could be Medicare or Medicaid recipients, and the plan had to be either a federally qualified HMO or based at a community health center that received federal funding from the Public Health Service. These restrictions, and a federal statute requiring that Medicaid recipients be free to choose their provider, limited the numbers of Medicaid recipients enrolled in managed care programs throughout the 1970s.

Omnibus Budget Reconciliation Act

In 1981, the Omnibus Budget Reconciliation Act (OBRA) granted states greater flexibility in structuring managed care arrangements for Medicaid beneficiaries. They were allowed to establish their own qualifications for HMOs serving Medicaid patients; and up to 75 percent of plan members (in an HMO that was contracting with Medicaid) could be Medicare and Medicaid enrollees. States were allowed to guarantee eligibility to Medicaid enrollees who wanted to join a federally qualified HMO. In addition, waivers of the freedom-of-choice provisions of the Social Security Act permitted states to establish primary care case management and to select Medicaid providers according to their cost-effectiveness.

Since the passage of OBRA, states have adopted two basic strategies in implementing managed care for Medicaid beneficiaries:

1. setting up primary care case management in which providers are either paid on a fee-for-service basis or, less often, on a capitated basis; and

2. organizing Medicaid programs in HMOs and reimbursing providers by capitation.

The passage of OBRA encouraged Medicaid beneficiaries to enroll in managed care programs. In June 1981, 282,000 Medicaid recipients were enrolled in prepaid health plans in 18 states. By December 1987, more than 1.5 million recipients had been enrolled by 31 states. HCFA estimates that, at present, about nearly 4 million people, or 13 percent of the nation's Medicaid recipients, are enrolled in managed care programs, and more are expected to be enrolled in 1995.

Current Federal Guidelines and Waivers

Today, managed care in Medicaid programs is restricted by federal law and allowed only under a special waiver granted by HCFA.[54] Section 2175 of OBRA 1981 enacted the freedom-of-choice waiver, which permits states to implement innovative approaches to providing care. States are able to receive waivers of certain program requirements—for example, the requirement that Medicaid recipients be free to select the provider of their choice. Several states have Medicaid demonstration waiver programs involving managed care, and more are expected in the near future.

In addition, Section 1115 of the Social Security Act authorizes experimental, pilot, or demonstration projects that, in the judgment of the Secretary of Health and Human Services, promote the objectives of Medicaid. Under this authority, HCFA can waive Medicaid requirements regarding amount, duration, and scope of services, as well as eligibility and reimbursement for services. HCFA also can waive requirements that all Medicaid services be statewide and that participants have freedom to choose providers. Many states have, or are applying for, such waivers in order to modify certain federal mandates as a way to experiment with cost-effective health care services to the poor.

Through July 1991, HCFA estimated savings from Medicaid managed care at almost $227 million. For example, a waiver program for substance abuse treatment in Minnesota saved an average of $3,500 per recipient over two years. A program for diabetes care in Maryland saved approximately $1,600 per recipient over two years. In South Carolina, a mental health case management program saved approximately $950 per recipient over two years.[55]

HMOs participating in the Medicaid program are required to limit Medicaid and Medicare recipients to no more than 75 percent of enrollees and to draw at least 25 percent of their enrollees from the private sector. This "75/25 rule" is imposed to ensure that care provided to Medicaid enrollees is comparable to that provided to enrollees with private insurance.[56]

Difficulties of Managed Care with Current Regulations

Because the U.S. population remains segregated by income, HMOs in a single locale find it difficult to serve both Medicaid and non-Medicaid patients with the same facilities; the 75/25 rule creates an operational barrier for health plans that wish to serve Medicaid populations but cannot enroll 25 percent through private insurance.

The Medicaid population presents certain other special needs that must be addressed by managed care organizations wanting to contract with a state. Those among the most critical are described below:

- Many Medicaid beneficiaries do not have primary care physicians or access to regular preventive care; they therefore often use the health care system inappropriately (e.g., expensive emergency room use for routine, nonemergency care).

- Medicaid beneficiaries are often in need of education and outreach services so that they learn to use the health care system in a cost-effective way.

- Medicaid beneficiaries frequently live in inner cities or rural areas, where access to managed care services is limited because those services have been geared toward a different demographic and geographic population.

- State Medicaid programs vary by benefit packages offered, target populations, reimbursement mechanisms, and the programs' voluntary or mandatory status for recipients, which makes it more difficult for a national or regional managed care organization to price services and provide services identical to their non-Medicaid-enrolled population.

Controlling Medicaid Managed Care

To address these issues, current Medicaid managed care programs use one or more of the control mechanisms described below.

Primary Care Case Management

Under this arrangement, a single provider is responsible for coordinating, arranging, and monitoring all the care a patient needs. The provider receives a flat case management fee. States may limit the number of Medicaid clients that a physician can serve in such a program.

Risk Contracts

States contract with HMOs or similar organizations to provide specified services in return for a predetermined fixed payment. The payment is based on the projected costs of a typical caseload. Federal rules require that this capitation rate be actuarially sound and not exceed the fee-for-service equivalent.

Comprehensive or Full Capitation Risk Contracts

Providers must offer at least three mandatory services under a Medicare risk contract and must agree to provide all other services mandated by Medicaid.

Partial Capitation Risk Contracts

Providers accept risk for a defined set of services (for example, physician services and either laboratory, x-ray, or clinic services). Other services are reimbursed on a fee-for-service basis. Records of payment are kept of the fee-for-service for each enrollee, and any savings are shared with the contractor.

Health-Insuring Organizations

These organizations assume an underwriting risk to pay for medical care provided to an enrollee in exchange for state-paid premiums. A health-insuring organization does not provide services directly,[57] but is a more traditional indemnity insurer.

Quality Requirements

Quality is an especially important issue for Medicaid managed care. Federal oversight (including freedom-of-choice provisions, the 75/25 rule, and the right of individuals to disenroll), annual quality review requirements, and state monitoring offer Medicaid enrollees quality safeguards. However, states argue that many of the federal requirements, especially the 75/25 rule, may hold Medicaid managed care to a higher standard than Medicaid fee-for-service arrangements.

Issues of Managing Medicaid Populations

In general, Medicaid fee-for-service rates and the capitation rates derived from them are considered by many to be unrealistically low, discouraging providers from participating in the system. This problem is compounded by the complexities of Medicaid eligibility. State welfare or Aid to Families with Dependent Children (AFDC) are often conditions for eligibility. When individuals on AFDC have a change in financial circumstances, they lose their eligibility to remain in the program. They also lose their Medicaid coverage and are disenrolled from their Medicaid HMOs. Medicaid HMO members may be enrolled in and disenrolled from the same plan several times a year, and many states are weeks or months in arrears in updating eligibility information, making the tracking of enrollment difficult.

With many states in financial crisis, legislatures are reluctant to increase their expenditures on Medicaid. Technical and regulatory barriers also hinder their attempts to implement an HMO-based strategy for Medicaid recipients. Nevertheless, several states have begun campaigns to increase Medicaid enrollment in managed care. For example, Arizona began its first Medicaid program in 1982 and, from the beginning, virtually all Medicaid eligible individuals were enrolled in managed care plans. New York passed a law in 1991 that seeks to enroll nearly 50 percent of the state's Medicaid eligibles in managed care within five years.

Expanding Managed Care to the Medicaid Population

The growth of managed Medicaid programs will, in part, depend on:

- the extent to which rate-setting mechanisms for managed care can be satisfactorily reformed;

- the elimination or modification of some demonstration project requirements that are impediments to experimentation;

- the elimination of the 75/25 rule; and

- welfare reform that will allow those who seek to get off welfare to keep health care benefits until they achieve some financial stability.

As in Medicare, managed care systems in Medicaid represent an opportunity to provide health care efficiently to a new population, but many barriers to service must be dealt with before such programs are common.

■ Military Health Services System

The Military Health Services System (MHSS) provides health benefits to more than 9 million active duty military personnel, retirees, their dependents, and survivors. Nearly 4 million of those enrolled in the MHSS are not active duty personnel.

Almost 10 percent of the beneficiaries in the MHSS are over 65 years of age, and that proportion will increase substantially in the future. The general aging of the military population is significant in terms of health care costs. Although health costs in the military have risen a little more slowly than in the civilian sector, there has been a 55 percent rise since 1985. The budget for MHSS medical operations in fiscal year 1991 was $15 billion.

In recent years, the Department of Defense has set up a number of demonstration projects to test the effects of cost and utilization controls. They are functioning within the MHSS Civilian Health and Medical Program of the Uniformed Services (CHAMPUS) program, which provides cost-sharing health benefits for the dependents and survivors of active duty personnel and for retirees and their dependents and survivors.

CHAMPUS benefit costs have almost doubled since 1985, and the number of claims under CHAMPUS more than doubled from 1985 to 1989. Clearly, CHAMPUS could benefit from cost management mechanisms.

CHAMPUS Reform Initiatives

The CHAMPUS Reform Initiative demonstrations include HMOs, POS plans, family practice and designated provider models, and PPOs, as well as a contracted provider arrangement for mental health care.

The demonstrations suggest that these models are effective in serving their members and in lowering costs. Patient satisfaction and cost savings were positive in the HMO and POS demonstrations. In California and Hawaii, the enrollment of 300,000 eligibles in HMOs and PPOs could save the Department of Defense an estimated $100 million over two years.[58] MHSS has been sufficiently impressed by these early results to incorporate many of the features of the demonstrations into a proposed Coordinated Care Program that will provide a rational system for health care delivery and financing.

■ Federal Employee Health Benefits Program

Managed care plans have been available to federal workers through the Federal Employee Health Benefit Program (FEHBP) for three decades. Originally, participation in HMOs by federal employees and their dependents was limited. In 1970, only 6 percent of all FEHBP beneficiaries had enrolled in an HMO.[59] However, buoyed by their limited experience with those plans, federal regulators were encouraged enough to support the HMO Act of 1973. The number of HMOs serving the federal plan grew from 21 in 1970 to 99 in 1980. By the end of 1991, more than 350 HMOs had enrolled 27 percent of the nearly 9 million FEHBP beneficiaries.[60]

From 1982 to 1992, the federal government commissioned several studies and held many hearings to examine methods of improving the government's health care programs. All recommendations for reform included suggestions that both the Office of Personnel Management (OPM) and Congress should apply the managed care alternatives found in the private sector to the government program. In particular, reform advocates recommended preadmission certification for nonemergency inpatient care, second surgical opinions, case management, and the increased use of HMOs and PPOs. OBRA-90 mandated several of these reforms, although OPM had already instituted the changes earlier that year. The changes forced all FEHBP fee-for-service plans to employ hospital precertification and case management. FEHBP beneficiaries who did not receive preadmission certification for nonemergency procedures would have their benefits reduced by $500.

Though legislation was proposed in 1991 to combine the many fee-for-service plans participating in FEHBP into one large federally sponsored plan, the Bush Administration opposed the bill because it was viewed as an increase to government costs, and the bill eventually died. However, some studies have estimated that similar reforms coupled with additional cost containment measures could save FEHBP between $200 million and $500 million annually.[61]

Although it is still too early to assess the cost savings effected by OBRA-90, FEHBP enrollees already are enjoying the improved quality measures offered by managed care. During the annual open enrollment period more than a quarter of FEHBP beneficiaries chose HMOs, and virtually all of the rest are enrolled in fee-for-service plans that are linked to PPO networks. It is hoped that, in the near future, the government health care program will resemble a private employer's triple option plan: an HMO, a provider network, and a POS option.

■ Other State Programs

Many state insurance programs have proved costly and difficult to manage. Managed care features or programs appear to be an effective way to address some of these issues. State government employee health benefit programs and workers' compensation programs are two of the major health insurance arrangements affecting state budgets, aside from Medicaid.

State Government Employee Health Benefits Programs

State government is usually a state's largest employer and, like other employers, state governments are turning to managed care for their employees. HMO and PPO participation varies widely among the 50 states. In 1992, 42 states made a total of 364 HMOs available to employees. Of the 3.6 million active employees covered by the 50 state plans, more than 1 million employees, about 30 percent, were enrolled in HMOs. Twenty-eight state health benefit plans offered a PPO. Of the 28, 20 used a POS plan in which the PPO was part of an indemnity plan; six states used PPOs with separate enrollment requirements; and two states incorporated both PPO types.[62]

In addition to participation in HMOs, most state employee health benefit plans have implemented cost management programs to help control indemnity plan expenditures. Almost half of all states have hospital inpatient precertification programs, concurrent review programs, and case management programs.[63]

■ Workers' Compensation Programs

Workers' compensation, established in 1911, is the oldest social insurance program in the United States. Every state has a workers' compensation law. Although similar in principle, no two jurisdictions have exactly the same benefits. Generally, the law applies to accidents and sicknesses that occur on the job.

Most states require that employers either obtain workers' compensation insurance by paying premiums for each worker, or give proof of financial ability to act as self-insurers.

Workers' Compensation Benefits

Several types of benefits are provided by the various laws:

■ death benefits to dependent survivors;

■ medical benefits for treatment of a sick or injured worker; and

■ loss of earnings benefits during total or partial disability, usually based on a percentage of wages.

Workplace injuries resulting in workers' compensation claims of long duration account for a large proportion of total costs of these laws. The national average cost of medical benefits per 100,000 workers in 1991 was almost $15 million ($150 per worker), up 11.8 percent from the comparable 1990 national average. Medical costs account for 40 percent of these benefit programs; they are the fastest-growing component of these charges.[64] Therefore, cost issues in the workers' compensation system mirror those being debated throughout the health care arena: access, financing, and reform.

State workers' compensation legislation focuses on strategies to reduce costs associated with workers' compensation. State legislatures are attempting to contain medical costs, reduce litigation, streamline administration, strengthen safety programs, and emphasize labor-management cooperation. The goal is to slow the growth of the rapidly rising costs associated with the workers' compensation system.[65]

Use of Managed Care Features

Workers' compensation programs are among the few remaining health insurance programs with little or no cost containment. Insurance carriers who managed workers' compensation accounts have made efforts over the past few years to institute some basic managed care features.

Hospital Utilization

Typical hospital utilization management techniques found in workers' compensation programs are precertification or prior authorization of nonemergency hospital admissions and concurrent review. These hospital utilization features help to reduce unnecessary admissions and lengthy hospital stays.

Case Management

Case management has become common in insurer-managed workers' compensation programs. The guiding principle of case management for large (catastrophic and costly) cases is to provide the highest-quality care in the most cost-effective manner possible. In fact, some managed care workers' compensation programs use case management techniques for all cases.

Because of an emphasis on providing a "holistic" approach to catastrophic cases, case management has been found to be a successful adjunct to workers' compensation programs and appears to have a positive effect on early return to work for beneficiaries.

Preferred Provider Organizations

A number of states have statutes that allow employers to designate providers for their employees' workers' compensation medical services, with allowance after 30 days for the employee to designate other providers. In those states, use is made of PPOs for medical services. As with the general population, once employees begin using PPOs, they rarely choose to go outside the plan.

PPOs have some difficulties in dealing with workers' compensation programs. Some problems are similar to those in PPO Medicaid programs, such as difficulty of having service providers conveniently available in the geographic area of the worker, and of workers having access to the type of care and providers needed for special medical needs.

Some insurance and managed care organizations have specifically targeted the workers' compensation industry by building networks that include the types of physician specialties that are critical to the treatment of occupational injuries.

Several states have attempted the challenging task of adapting workers' compensation programs to managed care principles of integrated services. At present, one difficulty of workers' compensation programs is integrating an employee's regular medical benefits with workers' compensation benefits. Several programs are described below.

24-Hour Coverage

Twenty-four-hour coverage has been defined by the National Association of Insurance Commissioners (NAIC) as "any combination of traditional health insurance and workers' compensation insurance that attempts to dissolve the occupational and nonoccupational boundaries between the two coverages."

Proposed 24-hour programs, though differing markedly from each other, generally fall into six basic types.[66]

24-Hour Coverage Marketing Program

This program offers coordinated or integrated management of workers' compensation and group health insurance claims. Most state laws do not allow combining the benefits available under workers' compensation with those available under other employee benefit plans. Therefore, these programs maintain separate policies and benefits, while integrating the services associated with the distinct policies (for example, billing, claims processing, medical management, disability management, and customer service).

24-Hour Medical Coverage

This approach provides medical benefits for all of an employee's injuries and illnesses, whether work related or not, while providing disability benefits for only those injuries or illnesses arising out of the job. A number of state legislatures have set up pilot programs that embrace this model.

24-Hour Disability Coverage

This approach provides disability benefits for all of an employee's injuries or illnesses while providing medical benefits for only work-related injuries or illnesses. This model was recommended by the New Jersey Commission on Income Maintenance in 1980, but the recommendations were never adopted.

24-Hour Coverage of Accidents

This approach provides medical and disability benefits for all accidental injuries and work-related illnesses; illnesses that are not occupationally triggered are not covered. An example of this approach is the New Zealand Accident Compensation system.

24-Hour Coverage of Diseases

This approach provides medical and disability benefits for all illnesses and work-related accidents; nonoccupational accidents are not covered. This design has been suggested in a number of contexts, but has yet to be implemented anywhere.

24-Hour Medical and Disability Coverage

This universal program provides medical and disability benefits for all injuries and illnesses, regardless of cause. The Netherlands provides this type of program to all employees.

Although the first program type outlined would maintain individual policies and retain benefit and coverage distinctions, the next five program types include consolidated or integrated policies and benefits. The impediments to this integration are substantial and include legal, institutional, and regulatory barriers. There has been much debate on the wisdom of resolving these obstacles. In the absence of consensus and the legislative changes necessary to move forward on the integrated coverage or benefit models, focus has shifted to the 24-Hour Marketing Program, or what is more commonly called 24-Hour Services.

The delivery of 24-hour service programs does not require enabling legislation, avoids most of the barriers that block delivery of the 24-hour coverage models, addresses the institutional issues that would need to be resolved for any of the models, and delivers most of the advantages of the coverage models.

24-Hour Services

Three variations of 24-Hour Service have emerged:

1. **24-Hour Medical.** Coordination of medical expenditures across occupational (workers' compensation) and nonoccupational (Group Medical) coverages.

2. **24-Hour Disability.** Coordination of disability expenditures across occupational (workers' compensation) and nonoccupational coverages.

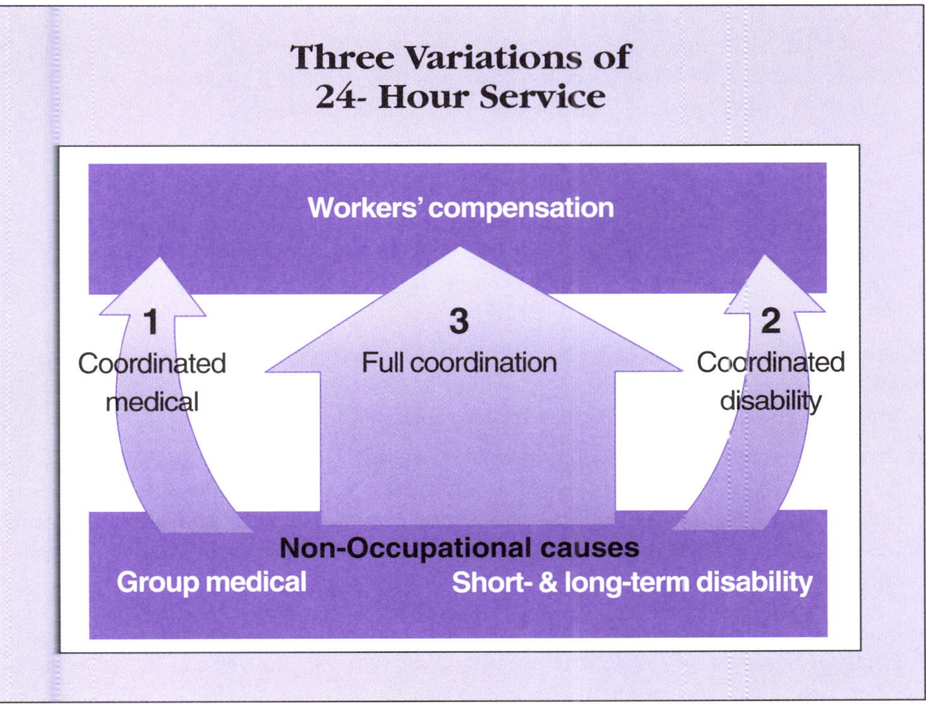

Figure 6.5

3. **24-Hour Medical and Disability.** Full coordination of both medical and disability expenditures.

(Figure 6.5)

Marketplace influences that have fueled the interest in 24-hour service include the growth of medical management in Workers' Compensation and the emphasis on disability management in health insurance. Medical and disability management services are equally applicable to occupational and non-occupational events.

Expected Benefits of 24-Hour Services

Consolidation of health and workers' compensation insurance allows:

■ **Administrative Savings.** Coordinated or consolidated services will cost less to administer than independently provided services.

- **Better Medical Management.** The coordination or consolidation of managed care techniques and services across an employer's total medical expenditures should result in increased consistency, network utilization, and the ability to apply medical management techniques sooner.

- **Administrative Simplicity.** An employer can do business with fewer suppliers.

- **Earlier Return to Work.** The coordination or consolidation of disability management techniques and services across an employer's total indemnity or loss of time expenditures should result in less time lost to disability and related expenses.

- **Avoidance of Duplicate Payments.** The coordination or consolidation of claims processing precludes the possibility of "double-dipping," or the payment of the same claim or loss by two policies.

- **Employee Simplification.** Employees must understand managed care programs in order for them to be most effective. Applying a single set of rules and procedures across multiple insurance or service plans simplifies the communication process and, therefore, maximizes both understanding and compliance.

A number of states have enacted legislation specific to 24-hour pilots. Although legislation is not required in any jurisdiction to enable the marketing of 24-hour service programs, the pilots are focusing public attention on these programs and allowing quantitative and qualitative evaluation of results. Going beyond anecdotal results to describe the anticipated benefits of these programs should greatly affect consumers' receptivity and interest in 24-hour coverage.

■ Managed Care Alliances

Several states have begun experimentation with managed care alliances. The purposes of these alliances is to enable small employers who have difficulty in affording insurance for their employees to expand their purchasing power. In addition, these alliances encourage the use of managed care principles and programs in their insurance pools to provide good-quality, cost-effective health plan benefits.

For example, in 1992, California enacted health alliance legislation that was part of small group market reform legislation. The Health Insurance Plan of California (HIPC), a voluntary alliance that became effective July 1, 1993, enrolled more than 3,000 employer groups with 54,000 enrollees in its first year. Approximately 72 percent of the groups used agent-broker services to enroll in the HIPC. Almost 23 percent of the employer groups were previously unin-sured.

The alliance is voluntary, which permits the small employer to determine on its own whether to purchase health coverage from the alliance, purchase coverage from an insurer outside the alliance, or purchase no insurance at all.

The Managed Risk Medical Insurance Board (MRMIB), which governs the program, developed the alliance's benefit design and determined that managed care was the most appropriate vehicle to offer comprehensive, cost-effective health care. Thus, by regulation, only HMO and PPO programs are offered through the alliance.

The MRMIB developed two benefit variations for each of the HMO and PPO products: standard and preferred. Although the scope of coverage is the same for each of the two products offered within the HMO or the PPO, the only variation between the standard and the preferred product is the copayment amounts paid by the individual. Thus, the premium for the preferred plan for both the HMO and PPO is greater than the corresponding standard plan because of smaller copayments.

The HIPC also is an employee choice program. Once the employer has made the decision to enter the HIPC and offer coverage to its employees, each employee chooses from the more than 20 (mostly HMO) health plans from which to obtain health coverage. Approximately 80 percent of enrollees participate in HMOs.

By statute, only four case characteristics permit rate variation: age, geography, benefit design, and family composition. Although the California small group reforms permit limited premium pricing variations for claims and health history, the HIPC does not permit any such price variation.

Other states have similar programs, with some variations. Florida's program, which became operational in 1994, permits, but does not require, exclusivity of managed care products in the 11 Community Health Purchasing Alliances (CH-PAs) The Texas program, which also became operational in 1994, permits any carrier in good standing (including HMOs) to participate. Kentucky's law restricts offerings to five standard plans, which may be offered as indemnity insurance or as an HMO. North Carolina's alliance, which becomes effective in 1995, requires two plans to be available, offered by two types of carriers: indemnity insurance and HMOs. Ohio's alliance program permits any insurance plan offered by an insurer, including an HMO, PPO, or any combination.

Rural Health Care Delivery Systems

Nearly 23 percent of the nation's population lives in rural areas, where there are shortages of physicians and adequate hospitals, low incomes, and small population. This creates significant problems in delivering and financing health care.

The National Rural Electric Cooperative Association (NRECA) reported that managed care plans are helping to improve health care availability and affordability in rural communities and concludes that managed care is growing in rural areas.[67] For example, the Interim Task Force on State Welfare and Medicaid Reform in Oklahoma has recommended that the Oklahoma Medicaid program be transformed into a comprehensive managed care system over the next five years. The task force noted that geography inhibits the organization of comprehensive health plans in some rural areas. In these areas, the task force suggests a primary care case management model, in which the state pays rural practitioners a fee to act as gatekeepers. Medicaid recipients would receive hospital and specialty care only if the primary care provider agreed it was necessary.[68]

■ Summary

Government, at all levels, is faced with issues of rising health care costs, inappropriate utilization of health care services, and problems of equity and access to health care. In an effort to address these problems, both the federal and state governments have attempted to incorporate managed care principles and programs into government-sponsored health care systems. Much experimentation is now occurring with regard to the best way to solve these problems in a high-quality and cost-effective manner. Insurers, managed care organizations, employers, and consumers all have a stake in government efforts to manage health care.

■ Key Terms

Adjusted Average Per Capita Cost (AAPCC)	Capitation rate	Competitive medical plans (CMPs)
Adjusted community rate (ACR)	Case management	Concurrent review
Aid to Families with Dependent Children (AFDC)	CHAMPUS Reform Initiative	Copayment
	Civilian Health and Medical Program of the Uniformed Services (CHAMPUS)	Cost basis
		Cost contracting
		Cost sharing
Capitation		Disenrollment

Duplicate payments
Federal Employee Health
 Benefit Program
 (FEHBP)
Federally qualified HMO
Fee-for-service
Financial risk
Fixed payment
Freedom-of-choice
 waiver
Full capitation risk
 contracts
Government Accounting
 Office (GAO)
Group Health
 Association of
 America (GHAA)
Health care prepayment
 plan (HCPP)
Health Insurance Plan of
 California (HIPC)
Health-insuring
 organizations
Health Maintenance
 Organization (HMO)
 Act
Hospital utilization
Indemnity plan
Independent Practice
 Association (IPA)
Integrated coverage
Integrated policies
Large (catastrophic)
 cases

Long-term care
Managed care alliances
Managed Risk Medical
 Insurance Board
 (MRMIB)
Medicaid
Medicare
Medicare Part A
Medicare Part B
Medicare qualified
 providers
Medicare SELECT
Military Health Services
 System (MHSS)
Network utilization
Nonemergency care
Office of Personnel
 Management (OPM)
Omnibus Budget
 Reconciliation Act
 (OBRA)
Overutilization
Partial capitation risk
 contracts
Partial disability
Point-of-service (POS)
 plan
Preadmission
 certification
Precertification
Preferred Provider
 Organization (PPOs)
Prepaid risk contract

Primary care case
 management
Prospective capitation
Risk adjustment
Risk contract
Second surgical opinions
Self-insurers
75/25 rule
Social Security Act
Tax Equity and Fiscal
 Responsibility Act
 (TEFRA) of 1982
Total disability
Traditional indemnity
 plans
Triple option plan
24-hour coverage
24-hour coverage of
 accidents
24-hour coverage of
 diseases
24-hour coverage of
 marketing program
24-hour disability
 coverage
24-hour medical and
 disability coverage
24-hour medical
 coverage
24-hour services
Waivers
Workers' compensation
 programs

Chapter 7

CONTROLLING QUALITY

117 *Introduction*

118 *Defining Terms*

119 *Quality Assurance*

122 *Treatment Protocols*

123 *Quality Assurance Studies (Problem Solving)*

125 *Continuous Quality Improvement/Total Quality Management*

134 *CQI Implementation*

135 *Benefits of CQI*

136 *Summary*

137 *Key Terms*

■ Introduction

What defines quality in health care? To a clinician, it may mean high immunization rates or low infant mortality rates. To a patient, it may mean less waiting time at a clinic. To an employer, it may mean the lowest price for basic benefit coverage.

The concept of quality in health care has grown and changed over the past few years as a result of increased medical costs, the evolution of managed care, the capacity to generate and store data, and the growth of significant competition among health care payers and providers. Traditionally, quality in health care meant using more technology, doing more tests, or delivering more intensive services, all of which tended to raise costs without demonstrable benefit. It was a definition of quality that sought to reduce defects even though it raised prices.

The demands of customers—patients and payers—to provide high-quality health care at a reasonable cost have shifted from a focus on the traditional model of quality to one focusing on systemwide, continuous quality improvement. The recent growth of managed care has helped foster this new environment because managed care combines the financing of health care with its delivery. A managed care organization can exercise greater control over the quality of health care by providing appropriate financial incentives.

Implementation of quality controls in managed care is critical to maintaining competitiveness in today's health care market. The quality provider will find it easier to gain and retain enrollees and contracts and will encounter fewer situations that could result in litigation. A high-quality, professionally managed health care network also will find it easier to recruit and retain high-quality physicians.

All stakeholders share involvement in the quality assurance process. Leaders among provider organizations use internal quality measures to maintain standards of quality. Regulators, as external stakeholders in managed care, have begun to use quality measures to monitor providers in an effort to maintain public standards. Payers for health care, who can be both external and internal stakeholders (patients, employers, government), use quality measures to compare the quality and cost of service from one provider organization to another.

This chapter examines the development of quality management in managed care, from the more traditional methods to the newer models, and the tools for continuous quality improvement.

■ Defining Terms

Understanding the concept of quality management in health care requires familiarity with several important terms and concepts. The important terms that will be used and explained in this chapter are listed below.

- **Consumer.** Users of health care services, such as patients getting care or providers getting support services from laboratories; payers of service, such as individuals, employers or the government; or the general public as beneficiaries of services.

- **Quality.** Meeting or exceeding customer expectations.

- **Quality Assurance (QA).** A set of activities that measures the characteristics of health care services and may include corrective measures.

- **Quality Improvement (QI).** Expands upon the concept of QA by using a proactive, prospective approach that is internally directed and focused on all persons and activities performed by the organization. QI, unlike QA, seeks to improve processes rather than merely solve problems.

- **Continuous Quality Improvement (CQI) and Total Quality Management (TQM).** Two terms, often used interchangeably, that describe a continual process of improving quality in the total health care organization. It is customer-focused and proactive. CQI seeks to prevent problems from occurring and, if problems do occur, to determine the underlying causes of the problem and then fix the process, not just the problem.

- **Outcome Measurement.** A tool, used to assess a health system's performance, that measures the outcome of a given intervention (e.g., death rates for a given procedure, days needed for recovery, etc.).

- **Outcome Management.** By using outcome measures, outcome management seeks to control and improve the quality of care and quality of medical outcomes through a continuous process.

- **Clinical Indicator.** A "measurable element in the process or outcome of care whose value suggests one or more dimensions of quality of care and is theoretically amenable to change by the provider."[69]

- **Practice Guideline.** A specific, professionally agreed upon recommendation for medical practice used within or among health care organizations in an attempt to standardize practice to achieve consistent quality outcomes. Practice guidelines may be instituted when triggered by specific clinical indicators.

- **Practice Standard.** Similar to a practice guideline, but is stricter and requires specific actions to be taken.

Quality Assurance

Health care providers use many processes and programs to achieve higher-quality services. Several have already been mentioned in previous chapters because they relate to provider controls that not only affect cost but also affect quality. The most common quality assurance control methods are listed below.

Financial Controls for Quality

For a number of years, insurers and providers have used a variety of financial incentives to improve quality and control costs. The most typical are listed below.

Hospital Privileges

Hospital privileges are the approved means by which physicians can provide care to their patients who have been hospitalized. A physician without hospital privileges cannot treat patients or be reimbursed for services. The threat of reduction, modification, or suspension of hospital privileges helps to ensure that providers in hospitals are conforming to accepted hospital practice parameters. A physician who is not allowed to work directly with his or her patients who are hospitalized will have reduced income. Reasons for reduction or suspension of privileges include excessive numbers of malpractice suits and overutilization of, or failure to conform to, accepted standards.

Withhold Arrangements

Withhold arrangements allow the managed care organization to assess efficacy of practice and utilization patterns and reward those providers who practice high-quality, cost-effective medicine. The withhold arrangement holds back a portion of payment until cost-effective, quality practice can be assessed. If provider practice has been effective, based on quality and cost expectations, part or all of the withhold will be released at the end of the year.

Denial of Payment

When services are deemed to be inappropriate, unnecessary, or of poor quality, payment may be denied. The insurer or payer will not pay for services that do not conform to benefit standards.

Clinical and Utilization Reviews

The utilization review process assesses quality of care as well as cost of care. Typical components of utilization review include:

- preadmission review or screenings for nonemergency hospital and surgical services;

- precertification or authorization screenings for medical referral or outpatient tests;

- retrospective (after-the-fact) reviews or screenings to determine patterns of utilization in relation to diagnosis;

- peer review and case audits which entail the retrospective review of medical encounters, case records, or medical notes;

- sentinel reviews of medical records based on triggers that suggest poor clinical outcomes; and

- concurrent review of utilization during the course of a hospitalization.

An examination of the utilization of services is an important component of quality control in a managed care organization. Managed care organizations measure the utilization of services against a set of criteria to determine the appropriateness and effectiveness of health care.

Credentialing

Credentialing, discussed in Chapter 3, is a method of reviewing a provider's previous work history, malpractice history, education, training, practice history, utilization, and medical board certification to determine if the person meets the selection criteria of the managed care organization.

Credentialing provides a practical objective focus for QA.[70] The data gathered for the credentialing process are used to determine whether or not a provider is a suitable candidate for the network. A thorough credentialing process entails the following elements:

- establishment of explicit standards and criteria from the managed care organization that define the goals of credentialing;

- verification of professional education, medical board examinations, and work history;

- analysis of practice patterns, including utilization and referral patterns;

- site review which, in the case of credentialing, is conducted in a potential provider office, clinic, or institution; and

- results of patient satisfaction surveys about provider service, when available.

Conducting most or all of these review activities in the credentialing and selection process will assist in developing or maintaining quality in a managed care network. Establishing and maintaining a sound credentialing process help to:

- reduce organizational risk, in that the managed care organization will have less chance of hiring impaired or substandard providers;

- increase the marketability of a managed care organization by enhancing the organization's reputation through its high standards;

- conform to quality standards of outside accrediting organizations for verification of credentials (accrediting by outside organizations is important for competitiveness and, in some cases, reimbursement for services); and

- maintain compliance with mandates by several states that managed care organizations conduct a credentialing process.

A thorough credentialing process involves not only the initial credentialing of providers, but also a recredentialing of providers (often every two years). The recredentialing process can include ongoing monitoring to alert the managed care organization to a change in compliance on the part of the participating provider.

■ Treatment Protocols

Development of treatment protocols is another way of enhancing quality in a health care organization. Treatment protocols are developed for clinical areas of medicine where diagnostic or therapeutic approaches are well defined. Technology assessment and quality studies are used to establish decision protocols for particular diseases or treatments. This quality process can be developed within a provider or managed care organization or can occur outside the organization (e.g., by a payer, through legal channels, or by other network organizations or provider groups).

Practice Guideline Development

Organizations with a large stake in the health financing and delivery system naturally have a major interest in the development of guidelines for practice. Thus, the interest of physicians, hospitals, insurers, medical specialty organizations, government agencies, and private organizations in the development of practice guidelines is not surprising. The American Medical Association (AMA) has endorsed the development of practice parameters. AMA's directory of practice parameters includes 1,600 listings of guidelines ranging from prenatal diagnoses to decisions near the end of life. The directory includes recommendations by 70 national physician organizations and several other groups.

One of the most important guideline development efforts began in 1989 with the creation of the Agency for Health Care Policy and Research (AHCPR) by the U.S. Department of Health and Human Services. Among its many responsibilities, AHCPR has used expert panels to develop guidelines for clinical practice.

The guidelines released by AHCPR through 1994 include:

- Acute Pain Management
- Pressure Ulcers in Adults
- Urinary Incontinence in Adults
- Cataract in Adults: Management of Functional Impairment
- Depression in Primary Care: Volume 1—Detection and Diagnosis; Volume 2—Treatment of Major Depression
- Sickle Cell Disease: Screening, Diagnosis, Management, and Counseling in Newborns and Infants
- Evaluation and Management of Early HIV Infection
- Benign Prostatic Hyperplasia: Diagnosis and Treatment
- Management of Cancer Pain

- Unstable Angina: Diagnosis and Management
- Heart Failure: Evaluation and Care of Patients with Left Ventricular Systolic Dysfunction
- Otitis Media with Effusion in Young Children.

Guidelines under development include:

- Acute Low Back Problems in Adults
- Quality Determinants of Mammography
- Recognition and Initial Assessment of Alzheimer's and Related Dementias
- Anxiety and Panic Disorders in the Primary Care Setting
- Smoking Prevention and Cessation
- Urinary Incontinence in Adults—Update
- Post Stroke Rehabilitation
- Cardiac Rehabilitation
- Screening for Colorectal Cancer

While the one goal of guidelines is cost-effectiveness, savings are not necessarily assured by their use. Some of the guidelines (such as those published by the AHCPR to establish appropriate treatment for sickle cell anemia) may, in fact, increase costs.

Guidelines can play an important part in the provision of quality services by eventually determining standards of practice. However, not every clinical situation can be managed by strictly adhering to a practice guideline. For example, overutilization of x-rays and electrocardiograms occurs not because of a lack of guidelines, but rather because of fear of litigation. Therefore, a quality practice environment necessitates more than merely developing practice guidelines.

■ Quality Assurance Studies (Problem Solving)

Many quality assurance activities parallel the steps in clinical management of a patient. Both approaches are problem-focused and use the problem-solving process to achieve higher-quality provision of services through more effective treatment. The clinical quality assurance process includes several steps.[71]

Setting Priorities

The first step in a quality assurance study is to select appropriate quality indicators. Among things to be considered are the types of problems involved, the importance of the indicator, the effectiveness and efficiency of current practice, and the feasibility and cost of achieving improvement.

Initial Assessment

The initial assessment stage of performing quality studies focuses on problem identification. Several different methods can be used to obtain evidence of the quality of clinical performance. Among the most common are:

- medical audits;
- chart reviews;
- indicator monitoring; and
- hypothesis testing.

These methods are generally retrospective in nature and allow an examination of previous actions and subsequent medical outcomes to assess quality.

One tool used in making the initial assessment is the acceptable standard of performance. Unless an acceptable standard of performance is determined, it is difficult to assess the need for improvement or the likelihood of success in instituting corrective action. Often, a clinical benchmark is used to make this determination. The benchmark is a point of comparison between desired outcomes and actual practice. For example, in the case of postoperative infection in heart bypass surgery, a benchmark may be set at 5 percent as the upper limit of allowable infection rates. A rate that is higher than 5 percent would be considered a less than acceptable standard of performance.

One important task in this initial assessment is to determine roles and responsibilities in the quality assurance process. Often, a quality assurance committee is appointed whose decisions determine actions to be taken within a specific timeframe. The committee assumes primary responsibility for corrective action and there is limited or no involvement by others in the organization.

Planning

Following the initial assessment comes the planning process that determines what suggested actions made by the quality assurance committee will be taken. A determination is made whether problems or deficiencies in quality are the result of poor assessment techniques or improper execution of the treatment plan.

124

Selection of Alternatives

The next stage of the problem-solving process is selection of alternatives. At this point, the alternatives identified are reduced to the single best approach, based on feasibility, cost, and practicality.

Implementation and Evaluation

At the appropriate time, action is taken to solve the problem. The results (outcomes) are measured and an evaluation is made to determine if the desired outcome has been achieved. There is ongoing monitoring to determine if any deviations from thresholds or standards occur. Follow-up action is taken if required.

Quality assurance activities may improve performance by identifying where or with whom the "fault" or problem lies. Because the traditional quality assurance problem-solving process is not systems-oriented, changes occur incrementally and only in relation to specific clinical situations.

■ Continuous Quality Improvement/Total Quality Management

CQI or TQM have become increasingly important methods for achieving and maintaining quality in managed care. Because managed care integrates the financing and delivery of health care in a systematic, customer-oriented, ongoing way, CQI has become a key method of achieving these goals.

CQI encompasses the elements of quality assurance and problem solving described above and expands upon these principles. Interest in quality improvement is the result of work by W. Edward Deming, who used this concept to help the Japanese rebuild their industrial capability after World War II. Deming's approach [72] relies on several important principles, listed below.

- To institute quality improvement, there must be commitment to the process at the highest organizational levels.

- The organization should be customer-focused, and customer should be defined broadly.

- A consistent, quality-oriented organizational purpose should be created, based on identification of actual and potential customers' needs.

- Ongoing feedback from processes and customer satisfaction should be used to achieve quality, not inspection (inspection is too late and unreliable).

- Systems of constant quality improvement should be developed, which in turn constantly decrease costs.

- On-the-job training should be instituted to ensure that all staff are able to perform their duties at the highest level of quality possible.

- Ongoing educational processes to enable continuous quality work should be developed.

- Competition between parts of an organization should be eliminated, and cooperation and "ownership" of common goals and purposes should be encouraged.

Deming's philosophy of quality is an interactive "chain reaction" with the following elements:

Deming's Chain

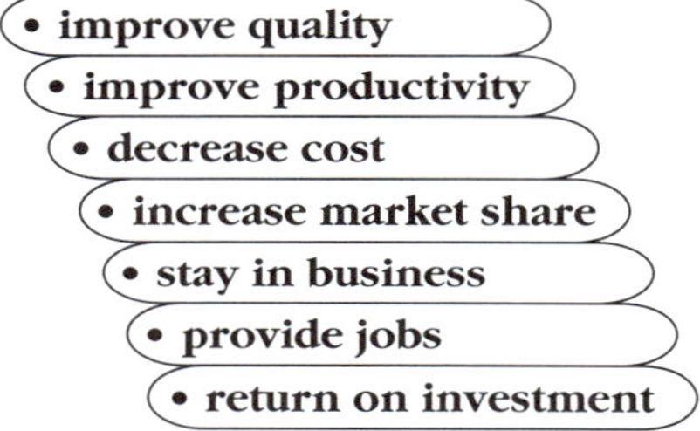

This chain reaction builds on systems theory that is based on the interrelatedness of all parts of an organization. Unlike the quality assurance approach, CQI's orientation is systemwide and continually occurring.

Differences between QA and CQI

The differences between QA and CQI are demonstrated in Figure 7.1.

Methods and Tools of CQI

In the CQI process, a wide variety of staff use methods and tools to examine the input, process, and outcome of activity. Much of the methodology is prospective. In addition to using the indicator monitoring technique of quality assurance (measuring elements of process or outcome to assess quality), the following are the most commonly used methods of CQI.

Comparison of QA and CQI

Quality Assurance	Continuous Quality Improvement
Goal of compliance:	Goal of meeting customer needs:
Customers are professionals and review organizations	Customers are patients, payers, professionals, review organizations
Generally retrospective, problem-solving orientation	Generally prospective, process-oriented
Static thresholds for quality indicators	Dynamic, continuous improvement
Few, specifically designated clinical staff involved in the process	All staff involved

Figure 7.1

Brainstorming

Brainstorming is a method for groups and teams to generate ideas about problems, possible causes, other solutions, and barriers to problem solving.

Affinity Analysis

This tool of problem solving makes use of the concept of brainstorming as a method of generating ideas, but takes the ideas generated by brainstorming and organizes them into affinities or relationship groups. This tool helps take the many ideas or pieces of information that are developed through brainstorming and categorizes them.

Systems Modeling

This technique is used to examine how various components work together (a so-called system) to produce an outcome. The most common way to conduct systems modeling is to diagram a model of the inputs, the process, and the outcome of a health care activity.

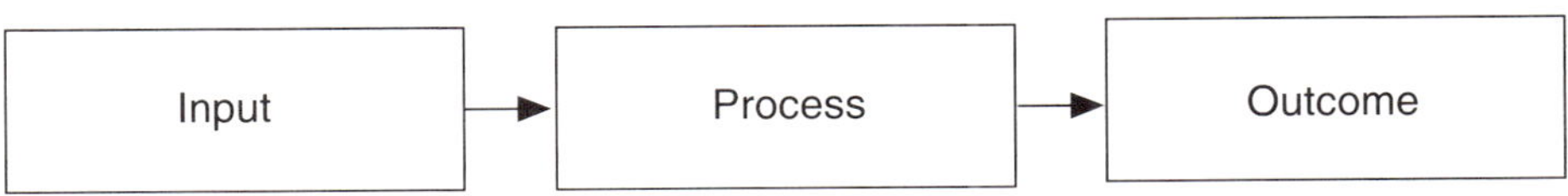

- Inputs are the resources needed to carry out an activity or process such as skilled labor, medications, and supplies.

- Processes are the activities and tasks that turn inputs into products or services such as conducting a physical examination, performing a surgical procedure, patient scheduling procedures, or taking a medical history.

- Outcomes are the result of processes and can be direct or indirect—an example of a direct outcome is the improved function of a joint following surgery to remove bone spurs. An indirect outcome would be patient satisfaction with waiting times at a clinic.

When identifying a major process or system that is to be modeled, a special concern is to determine the impact of the process. Examining impact (e.g., a significant reduction in cost or significant reduction in waiting time for 50 percent of all patients) is an important consideration in modeling. Quality improvement is served best when system models are based on important or high-impact areas. When developing a modeling process, it is often good to work backwards from the impact to conduct the analysis.

Flow Charts

A flow chart is a graphic presentation of how a process works, often by showing a sequence of steps. Flow charts help to present current processes, areas for improvement or increased efficiency, and key elements of the process, such as important areas for monitoring or data collection. In addition, flow charts are used to identify appropriate team members, determine who provides inputs or resources, and allow development of hypotheses about causes of problems.

There are several different kinds of flow charts. The key elements of each identify the process of creating outputs. Each chart includes inputs, steps, and product.

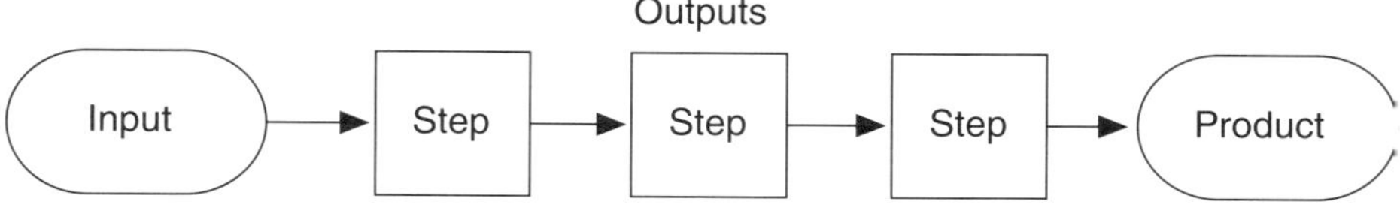

Some flow charts can be more detailed, but contain the same elements as the simple flow chart design described above. For example:

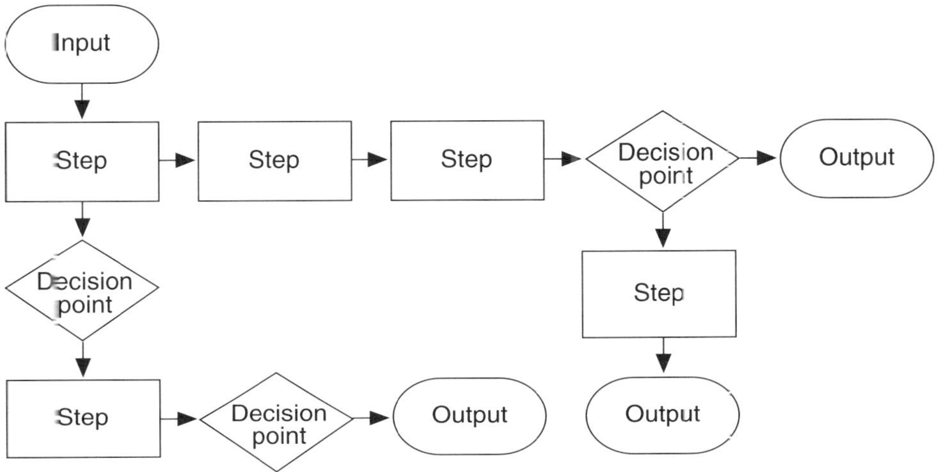

This type of flow chart is useful to examine areas of a process in detail and to look for problem areas or inefficiencies.

Regardless of the type of flow chart, several steps are used in its construction.

- Define the purpose of the chart and the format that is most appropriate.
- Determine the beginning and end points of the process to be charted (What are the inputs? How do we know when the process is complete? What are the final outputs?).
- Identify the elements of the flow chart (Who provides the input for a given step? Who uses it? What decisions need to be made? What is the output of a step?).
- Reflect what actually occurs in a process, not an ideal.
- Focus the chart on identified problems.

Cause-and-Effect Analysis

Cause-and-effect analysis, which helps a team's brainstorming process, is depicted by two different graphic methods—the fishbone diagram and the tree diagram.

Fishbone diagram. The fishbone diagram, so called because of its shape, was developed by Kaoru Ishikawa to determine an effect (either desirable or undesirable) produced by a system of causes:

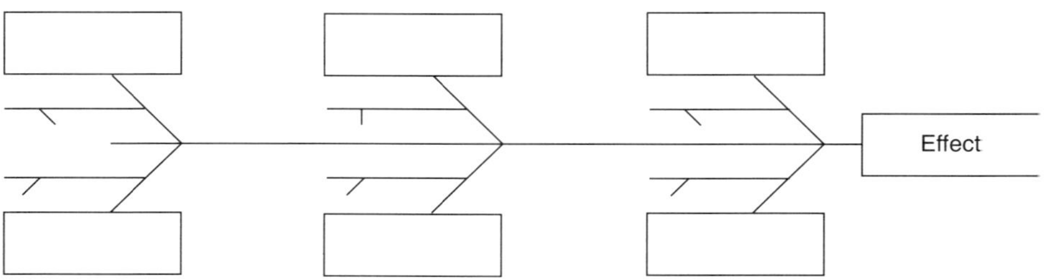

In the cause-and-effect diagram, brainstorming input should be provided by a variety of persons involved in a process. An effect (outcome) is determined, and the group then brainstorms to come up with the most complete and realistic causes (or inputs) that create this effect.

Tree diagram. The tree diagram highlights a chain of causes by grouping or categorizing a branching effect. It displays the layers of causes and assists in looking in depth for the root cause or causes of a problem.

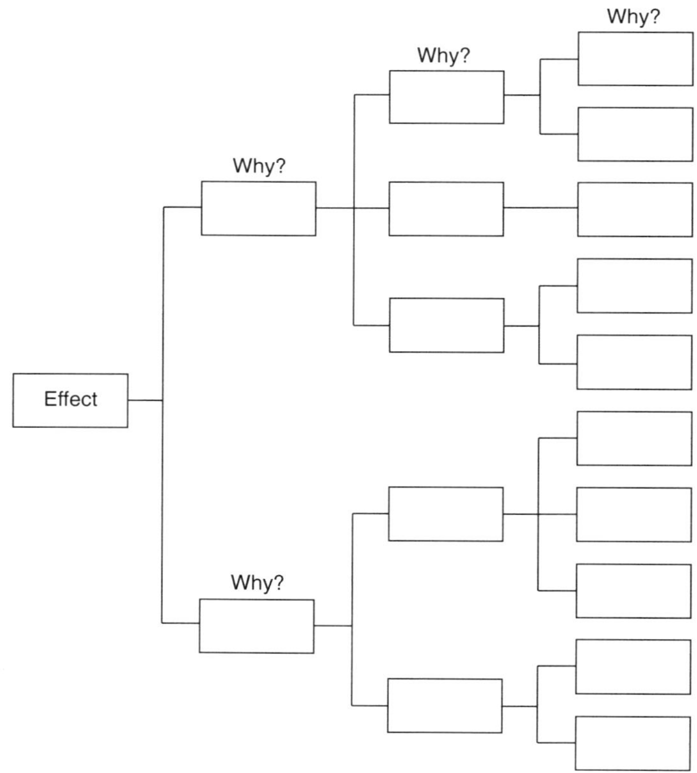

All cause-and-effect diagrams hold several elements in common:

- define the problem or desired outcome in the effect box;
- define the major steps or categories of input;
- identify specific causes;
- keep asking "why?" and
- check the logic of the chain of causes.

When this process is complete, it is often a wise idea to reduce the list of causes to simple forms in order to develop simple data collection tools to prove the theory or the cause.

Bar and Pie Charts

Bar and pie charts, which compare different groups, present data as a picture that allows the results to stand out. Bar charts generally are used to sort data into categories or divide data within each category. Examples of two kinds of bar charts are found below:

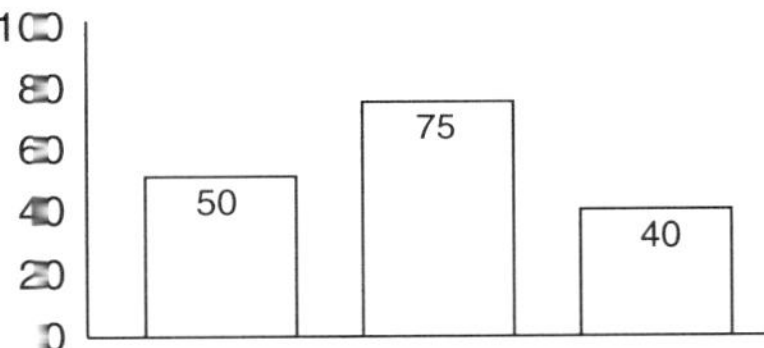
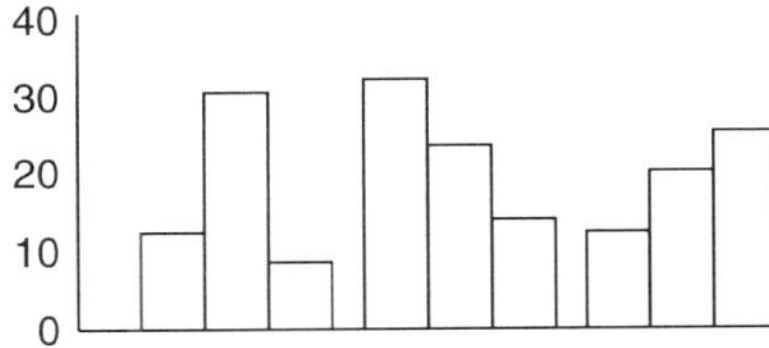

The pie chart categorizes data and calculates the percentage contribution for each element or factor under consideration:

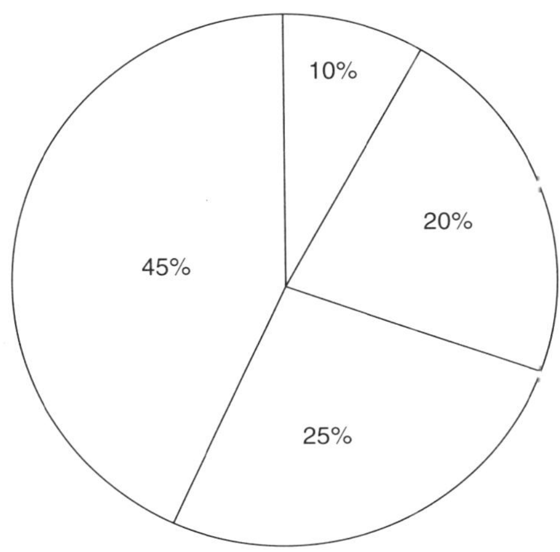

Charts must use scales at regular intervals, in an effort not to mislead the viewer. When charts are used to compare data, the comparisons also must be on the same scale.

Scatter Diagrams

Scatter diagrams give a picture of association between two variables. They can point to, though not prove, a causal relationship, or they can indicate that there is no causal relationship. A strong correlation (suggestions of causal relationship) is shown in example (a) and a weak correlation is shown in example (b). Example (c) shows no correlation and would indicate that the cause suggested for a particular outcome was not correct.

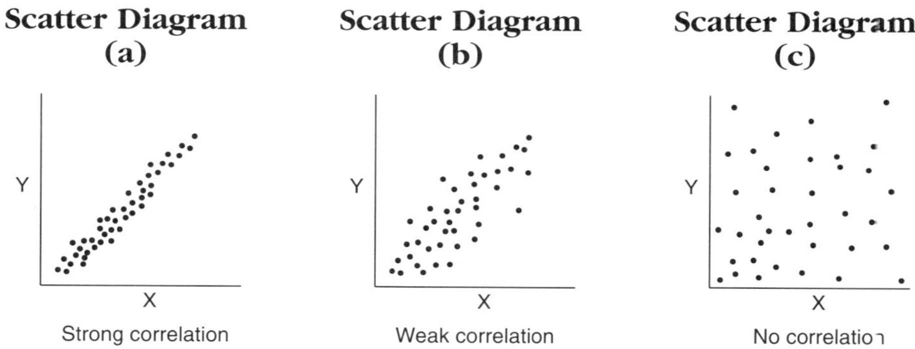

Gantt Charts

Gantt charts provide graphic presentations of how to carry out a series of steps in a quality improvement process. These charts are very useful in the planning process because they allow the user to understand what tasks must be carried out and the linkages between and timing of activities.

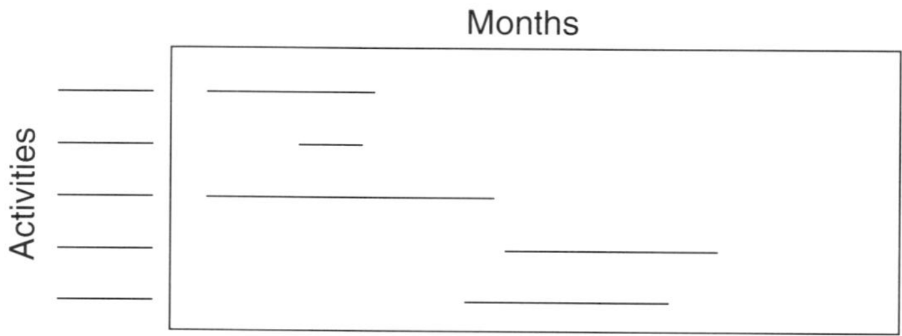

Pareto Chart

The Pareto chart organizes and displays information that can show the relative importance of various problems or causes of problems. The Pareto chart is a special form of a vertical bar chart that ranks items from highest to lowest order of importance. The basic principle of the Pareto chart is that whenever many factors affect a situation, only a few factors will account for most of the impact. By placing the items in descending order of importance, it is easy to discern those causes or problems that have the greatest effect on an outcome. In order to improve the quality of a given process, the Pareto chart helps to focus activity and thinking on those factors that have the greatest impact and prevent spending time and effort on relatively unimportant factors.

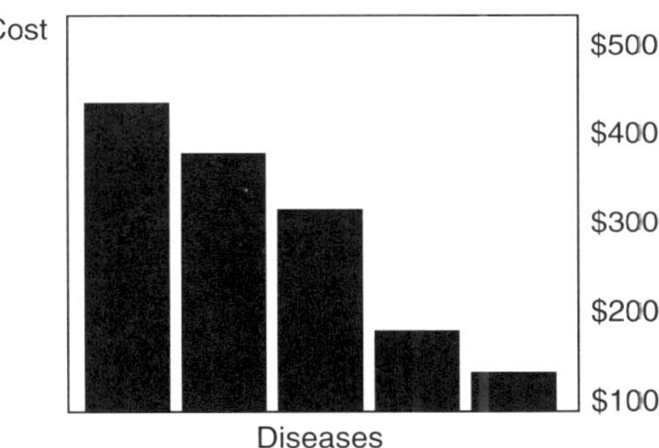

Developing the Pareto chart involves the following steps:

- developing a list of problems or causes to be compared;
- developing a standard measure for comparison of items (e.g., frequency of occurrence, amount of resources used);
- choosing a timeframe to collect all data; and
- listing all data collected in decreasing numerical order to create the chart.

Benchmarking

Benchmarking is a quality measurement tool that takes information from others' successes in an area where quality improvement is needed. In developing solutions to quality problems, it is helpful to gain knowledge of how others are approaching the same situation. It also is helpful to use benchmarking to identify areas of improvement by understanding the level of quality others have been able to achieve.

An example of benchmarking is the development of rates or percentages of less than optimal quality outputs. For example, your HMO has an average waiting time for appointments of 35 minutes, whereas the regional average waiting time for other HMOs is 15 minutes. You may wish to set your benchmark level at 15 minutes and then assess the inputs and steps needed to achieve the benchmark. It is important, when using benchmarking, that the process being considered is well understood and applicable to your organization.

■ CQI Implementation

A number of models are used to implement CQI. One of the most popular models in use by health care organizations is FOCUS-PDCA, developed by the Hospital Corporation of America in 1989.[73] This process, unlike the QA studies/problem-solving model, is process-oriented and continuous in nature.

FOCUS-PDCA

(F) ind	Who is the customer? What process needs improving? Who will benefit from improvement?
(O) rganize	Who and how many are on the team? Does the team have knowledge of the process?
(C) larify	Is the process defined clearly? Is there agreement on the best method for action?
(U) nderstand	How did the team identify process variables? Is there understanding of process variation? Is there a data collection plan?
(S) elect	What were the team's criteria for making a selection of method for change?
(P) lan	Does the team have a plan for improvement? Does the team have a plan for collecting needed data?
(D) o	How was the plan executed? Did the team collect data appropriately? Did the team analyze the data collected?
(C) heck	Did the data change? Was the process improved? Is the team comfortable with the data collected?
(A) ct	What did the team learn? Can the team continue using this process?

Figure 7.2

The FOCUS-PDCA model for implementing process change, and others like it, seek to find a process to change, assemble a team that knows the process, identify customers and the process outputs that meet customer needs, gather accurate data, analyze the data, document the process, eliminate inappropriate variation, and document continuous improvement.

FOCUS-PDCA is a process that continually asks questions that are important to health care organizations. These questions typically include:

- What are we trying to accomplish?

- How will we know that a change is an improvement?

- What changes can we make that we predict will lead to improvement?

- How shall we plan a pilot test?

- What are we learning as we do the pilot?

- What have we learned as we check and study?

- What needs to be done as we act to hold the gains or abandon our pilot?

The PDCA portion of the model, a continuous process that is pictured below, makes extensive use of data. (Sources of data are described in Chapter 8.)

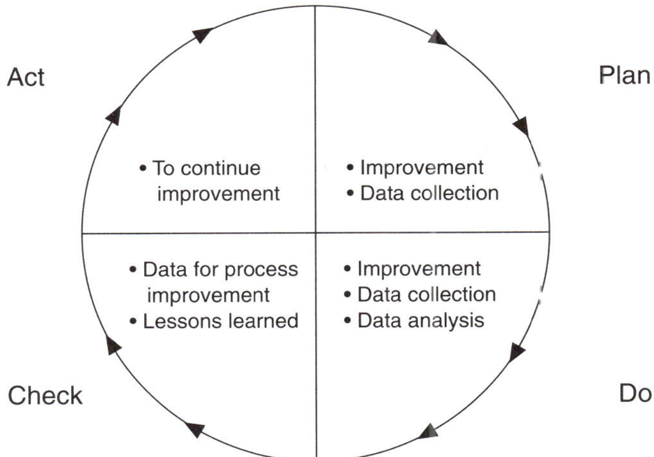

■ Benefits of CQI

CQI is not an easy method to implement. It takes commitment and work to develop an ongoing program of process improvement. However, there are numerous benefits for a managed care organization in implementing CQI.

Customer Satisfaction

The CQI process is customer-focused. As described earlier, customer is defined very broadly in managed care. Customers can be network providers, patients, enrollees, contractors, payers, employers, and the community. CQI demands that all customers be identified and their needs assessed. In addition, enrollee satisfaction surveys and focus groups are used to determine whether the outputs or outcomes of the CQI process are actually meeting identified needs.

Professional Quality Improvement

Implementing CQI can be a source of conflict for medical professionals who have practiced in the traditional, autonomous manner. CQI places responsibility for outcomes on the processes of the entire system, rather than on one individual. In managed care, clinical professionals must be accountable for both outcomes and process performance on a continuing basis. Therefore, the CQI process is ideal for instituting continuous clinical quality of practice.

Productivity Improvement

The focus on continual monitoring and improvement of process in CQI leads to improved quality outputs. The Deming chain reaction (above, p. 126) demonstrates that improved quality also decreases costs. Through analysis and making systems inputs more effective, quality of outputs is improved. By way of example, if through the CQI process a more efficient method of scheduling Magnetic Resonance Imaging is developed, more patients can be screened per day with the same number of personnel and amount of equipment. Higher-quality, efficient outputs will result in lower overall costs.

■ Summary

Managed care organizations seek to provide the highest-quality care for the lowest possible cost. They expect that the financing and delivery of health care services work in concert to achieve this goal. There are numerous ways that managed care organizations attempt to achieve cost-effective, quality service, including utilization controls, management analysis tools, quality assurance, and quality improvement methods.

Those managed care organizations that are least developed generally use retrospective methods of assessing quality. The more highly organized and controlled managed care organizations use more prospective, continuous methods of achieving high standards of quality.

■ Key Terms

Affinity analysis
Agency for Health Care
 Policy and Research
 (AHCPR)
American Medical
 Association (AMA)
Authorization
Bar charts
Benchmark
Benchmarking
Brainstorming
Case audits
Causal relationship
Cause-and-effect analysis
Clinical indicator
Concurrent reviews
Continuous Quality
 Improvement (CQI)
Correlation
Cost-effectiveness
Credentialing
Customer focus
Customers
Deming's chain reaction
Denial of payment

Fishbone diagram
Flow charts
Focus groups
FOCUS-PDCA
Gantt charts
Guidelines for clinical
 practice
Hospital privileges
Impact areas
Input
Malpractice
Medical board
 examinations
Outcome
Outcome management
Outcome measurement
Overutilization
Pareto chart
Patient satisfaction
 survey
Peer review
Pie charts
Practice guideline
Practice parameters
Practice patterns

Practice standard
Preadmission review
Precertification
Process
Quality
Quality assurance (QA)
Quality improvement
 (QI)
Recredentialing process
Referral patterns
Regulators
Retrospective
Retrospective reviews
Scatter diagrams
Sentinel review
Site review
Standards of care
Technology assessment
Total quality
 management (TQM)
Treatment protocols
Tree diagram
Withhold arrangements

Chapter 8

DATA FOR QUALITY, COST, AND UTILIZATION CONTROL

139 *Introduction*

140 *Sources of Data*

140 *Relation of Data to Time*

141 *Types of Managed Care Information*

142 *Other Calculations and Data*

144 *Automated Systems in Health Care*

145 *Management Information Systems*

145 *Types of MIS Systems*

147 *Controlling Fraud and Abuse*

150 *Data for Behavioral Health Management*

151 *Data for Outcome Measures*

151 *Data Requirement of Certifying or Accrediting Organizations*

154 *Summary*

155 *Key Terms*

■ Introduction

The systems modeling concept of INPUTS-PROCESS-OUTPUTS described in Chapter 7 requires information and feedback. Data are needed to understand what inputs or resources are available as well as to measure process and output. The feedback process of continuous quality improvement necessitates an ongoing infusion of data to analyze current operations. The model below demonstrates the relation of information and feedback to the elements of systems modeling.

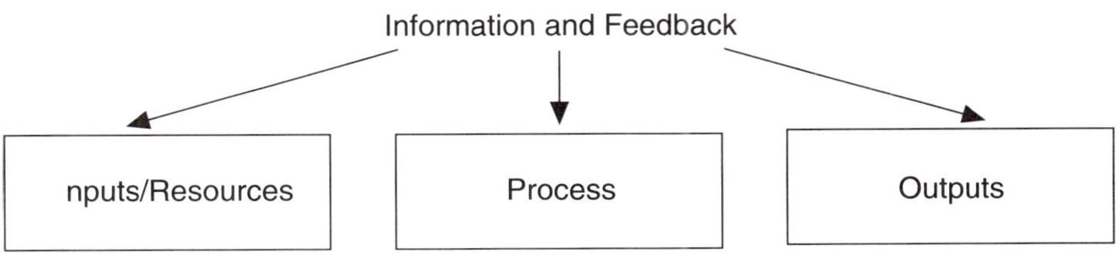

The types of data most helpful in managed care are those that help define clinical quality, acceptability of services to payers and patients, and accessibility of services. This chapter considers the many types of data, information, and measurements that can assist in controlling quality, cost, and utilization in health care organizations.

■ Sources of Data

The data needed to measure quality, cost, and utilization can come from a wide range of sources, both internal and external to the managed care organization. Frequently used data sources include:

- medical records;

- encounter data;

- case samples;

- physician profiles;

- patient questionnaires and interviews;

- products of utilization review processes;

- claims;

- data about facilities, equipment, and supplies (e.g., inventories and purchase orders); and

- comparative measures from outside organizations and groups (such as consumer report cards).

■ Relation of Data to Time

It is important to consider the time value of data in order to use them effectively to make comparisons or to judge effectiveness of outcome. Data are most frequently measured on a yearly, a seasonal, or a monthly basis. Data gathered for similar time periods should be used for comparison.

Time also is a factor when determining the fixed period under consideration for data gathering. In clinical measurement, this may be a period of hospitalization or an episode of illness. Care must be taken in defining time parameters because individual variation can exist at the beginning and at the end of any episode of care.

■ Types of Managed Care Information

Certain common ratios and statistics are used regularly to measure the effectiveness of a managed care organization. These calculations are developed from a variety of data. The most common of these calculations are listed below.

Per Member Per Month

This computational designation for each enrollee in a managed care program is commonly abbreviated as PMPM.

Cumulative Member Months

Cumulative Member Months (CMMs) are used extensively in calculating indicators and rates of occurrence. These indicators and rates in managed care depend heavily on PMPM data to control costs or determine capitation rates. CMMs are calculated in the following manner (Mbrs = members, and Mo = month):

$$\Sigma \ (MbrsMo1) + (MbrsMo2). . . = CMM$$

Per Member Per Year

Services per member per year (PMPY) is a mathematical figure that can be used to estimate and compare utilization rates of different primary care physicians or medical groups within a network. Rates can vary depending on the type of services being examined. For example, the normal HMO PCP may have three to four visits per member per year, but a pediatrician may see the average newborn to one-year-old seven times in one year. The calculation of services PMPY is as follows:

$$\frac{\text{Total Services} \times 12}{\text{CMM}} = \text{Services PMPY}$$

Cost Per Member Per Month

This measure is useful in comparing costs of different providers and services. The formula divides the total cost for services (e.g., office visits, x-rays) in the period being examined by the CMM for the period.

$$\frac{\text{Cost of Services}}{\text{CMM}} = \$PMPM$$

Hospital Days per 1,000 Enrollees

This calculation allows for comparison of hospital utilization by PCPs, specialty groups, medical groups, employer groups, patient groups, and managed care organizations. Often, hospital days per 1,000 enrollees is calculated monthly. The total hospital days in any given period are multiplied by 12,000 and divided by CMMs.

$$\frac{\text{Hosp Days} \times 12 \times 1,000}{\text{CMM}} = \text{Days/1,000}$$

Financial Performance

Assessing financial performance of a managed care organization is extremely important in making management and clinical decisions as well as in demonstrating to regulators, accrediting bodies, and payers that it is a solvent, efficient organization. Some of the more common rates and formulas for assessing financial conditions in managed care are listed below.

Common Ratios

$$\frac{\text{Physician Expenses}}{\text{Member Months}} = \text{Physician Expense PMPM}$$

$$\frac{\text{Hospital Expenses}}{\text{Member Months}} = \text{Hospital Expense PMPM}$$

$$\frac{\text{Other Medical Expenses}}{\text{Member Months}} = \text{Other Expenses PMPM}$$

$$\frac{(\text{Premium Revenue}) - (\text{Health care Expenses})}{\text{Member Months}} = \text{Gross Margin PMPM}$$

$$\frac{\text{Net Income}}{\text{Revenue}} = \text{Profit Margin}$$

$$\frac{\text{Total Incurred but Not Reported (IBNR) Claims}}{\text{Total Members}} = \text{Total IBNR per Members}$$

■ Other Calculations and Data

Other calculations commonly used are outpatient forecasting and profiling.

Outpatient Forecasting

As managed care evolves, many hospitals are developing comprehensive out-patient programs. This entails designing, constructing, and staffing outpatient surgery centers, walk-in clinics, and medical offices. Not only do developers have to decide what hospital services can be shifted to ambulatory care, but they must assess whether those services will increase patient volume and generate additional revenues.

To assist in strategic planning for outpatient services, a number of organizations have turned to database forecasting. Outpatient forecasting databases use in-patient data to estimate utilization in a hospital market. In addition, they attempt to predict future patient volume for certain hospital procedures within the market being considered.

Profiling

The concept of profiling—gathering data in order to compare practice patterns among physicians—is an increasingly common measure of quality in managed care. In fact, managed care organizations have taken the lead in this type of data gathering because they are so involved in affecting medical practice patterns and the quality outcome of practice.

Profiling is a systematic method of collecting, collating, and analyzing patient data to develop provider-specific profiles. Information about patient risk factors may be used to analyze the data, such as patient's age, diagnosis, and functional status. Often, however, risk factors do not account for the unexplained variation in medical practice. For example, the Maine Medical Assessment Foundation (MMAF) found a threefold variation in hysterectomy rates in different parts of the state of Maine. It was determined that the varying rates gave no significant difference in outcome, and the variation was unexplained. Through a feedback process of information to obstetricians and gynecologists, hysterectomy rates in the study areas dropped to the state average of two per 1,000 population.[74]

Data sources for profiling need to be reliable and up to date in order to make the best use of profiling. Data also must be available to understand why variations exist. Included among the most common data sources for profiling are:

- claims data;

- encounter data;

- admissions data;

143

- patient clinical records; and

- utilization data (both patient- and provider-specific).

Data elements that are used in profiling include:

- hospital admission and readmission rates;

- enrollee-specific encounter rates; and

- clinical indicators such as infection rates, immunization rates, death rates, and birth rates.

Unfortunately, these common sources of data may not be as useful as desired. For example, claims data is gathered primarily for billing purposes and does not usually capture relevant clinical details. Also, clerical errors and other inaccuracies can occur in coding claim forms, making the data obtained less sound.

Because of problems with traditional data sources, other data have been used for profiling, including administrative files and laboratory reports. However, it is difficult and often expensive for one managed care organization to capture accurate and necessary data to create accurate profiles. Therefore, several profiling programs have been developed to link data gathering and data-gathering systems in geographic areas, among all providers in a managed care network, or by government payers.

In the case of government payers, the Health Care Financing Administration conducts some profiling activities on a nationwide basis for Medicare beneficiaries. Medicare physicians can receive comparative reports on services provided per 1,000 Medicare beneficiaries.

Those managed care organizations that do profiling view it as a part of continuous quality improvement and as an excellent way to control utilization. While profiling should not be used in a punitive way, it can be used to inform physicians of how their practice patterns compare with those of other physicians and what changes they should make. Sanctions for providers whose profiles are outside acceptable ranges can include education, reductions in pay, limitations on reimbursement, or, in some cases, dismissal from employment or participation in the network.

■ Automated Systems in Health Care

In the past decade there has been increasing awareness of the need for health care information that encompasses the entire community rather than separate organizations. The community includes all organizations involved in generating, providing, accessing, or processing health care data related to physicians, hospitals, pharmacists, laboratories, dentists, payers, banks, and purchasers of health care services.

Automated systems in the health care setting can generally be classified into two categories: administrative and clinical. Administrative systems in hospitals and physicians' offices provide services in administrative areas such as patient registration, scheduling of appointments, accounting, accounts payable, purchasing, and inventory management.

Administrative systems for payer organizations provide automated services for functions such as claims adjudication, premium collection, customer service, and policyholder and provider reporting. Clinical systems provide services for functions including laboratory test processing, radiology (x-rays), and the ordering of medical procedures and tests for patients.

■ Management Information Systems

Managers of health care organizations rely on data and information in order to plan, solve problems, and control costs, utilization, and quality. It is extremely important for them to gain timely, accurate, complete, and appropriate information. The most efficient method of doing this is through management information systems (MIS).

MIS is a term used to describe computer systems that gather, store, and report information as needed. Traditionally, such systems were developed in-house, but over the past decade administrative and clinical systems for health care organizations have begun to be developed by hundreds of software companies. In the United States today, there are hundreds of administrative systems for physician offices, hospitals, and payers.

■ Types of MIS Systems

These information systems, some of which are highly sophisticated, generally are of three types: applications reporting systems, database management systems and decision support systems (DSS). The more sophisticated DSS systems will allow statistical simulation so that questions can be asked or projections can be made. For example, an interactive DSS system can be asked to project the economic effect of adding a 30 percent increase in Medicare Risk contract enrollees to the current enrollee base of an HMO.

There are a number of areas in a managed care organization that may be served by MIS systems. The main ones are clinical quality assurance and quality improvement, cost control and productivity management, utilization analysis and control, budgeting, planning, and evaluation.

Clinical Quality Assurance and Quality Improvement

The clinical information that is taken from patient records is now being computerized. Data are entered directly or are transcribed from written notation into the computer system. These data are processed into reports that allow peer review committees, quality assurance committees, quality improvement teams, and clinical managers to assess practices and clinical outcomes. They can be used as a basis for corrective actions when outcomes are not at expected levels of quality.

Cost Control and Productivity Management

Computerized systems allow for cost analyses and productivity reports that can be used by management for improving the efficiency and cost-effectiveness of managed care operations. For example, data on cost of magnetic resonance imaging (cost of equipment, staff, and space) divided by frequency of use will allow a health organization to:

- assess the costs of one test;
- determine if equipment and staff are used productively; and
- suggest possibilities for more cost-effective scheduling of tests.

Utilization Control and Analysis

Complete, well-designed information systems should contain both current and historical data on utilization of health services within a managed care system. The efficiency of resource utilization can be examined using these data to improve quality and change resource allocation and use. The example of magnetic resonance imaging above would allow data to be used to analyze effective utilization of the equipment.

Demand Analysis

The data gathered for utilization analysis can be used to assist managed care organizations in predicting demand for resources and services in the future. From data systems, trends can be discerned that help determine allocation of resources to provide quality services to internal and external customers.

146

Planning and Evaluation

The data captured through various MIS system applications outlined above, combined with demographic data, can also serve management in evaluation of current programs, projecting future service needs, and planning for development of new services and programs.

Other MIS Uses

As can be seen, MIS play an important role in all aspects of managing high-quality, cost-effective health care organizations. Organizational systems have been demonstrably effective in assessing workflow, processes, procedures, problem identification, reporting, and outcome measurement. The data available through MIS also can have a positive impact on customer relations by:

- providing the necessary claims and utilization information to customer service representatives of a managed care organization;

- controlling processes that lessen the likelihood of appeals and adjustments of claims;

- monitoring and enhancing quality, thereby improving customer satisfaction;

- lowering risk of litigation through effective documentation and monitoring of processes and procedures; and

- enhancing provider relations by providing useful and timely reports and reimbursement to providers.

■ Controlling Fraud and Abuse

Fraud and abuse in managed care, as in other types of insurance, are a reality and can inflate the cost of providing health care services. The types of fraud seen under fee-for-service reimbursement have been associated with incentives to overutilize services and incentives to seek reimbursement for services that might not have been provided. Under managed care, especially capitated payment arrangements, there are incentives to commit the following types of fraud:

- submission of false or misrepresented cost data in order to obtain a higher capitation rate;

- registration of fictitious enrollees;

- deliberate failure to provide necessary services; and

- payment of kickbacks for referrals of certain types of patients.

147

Management information systems are invaluable tools to detect and control fraud and abuse. Many data tools are used to enhance security. To do this, triggers or "red flags" have been developed to control medical fraud and abuse.

MIS systems offer opportunities to improve detection of health care fraud by generating more comprehensive and standardized data in which fraudulent billing patterns might be detected. Automated systems can facilitate the review of data that cannot otherwise be easily analyzed. There are two general approaches to analyzing health care fraud data: retrospective and prospective. Retrospective data analysis involves reviewing large amounts of historical information to identify patterns of fraudulent behavior. Prospective data analysis involves analyzing current data on a case-by-case basis, such as claims submitted but unpaid, and determining if the claim is legitimate and should be paid.

It is necessary to perform retrospective analyses of claims history to determine patterns of behavior and identify trends that are potentially fraudulent. Prospective techniques include evaluation of submitted claims to delay or prevent payment of suspicious claims. The suspicious claims can be flagged for more careful scrutiny, and legitimate claims can continue through for processing. Prospective utilization review (described in Chapter 7) can identify questionable service before it is rendered.

Some health care organizations have developed their own automated tools to assist in fraud detection. The most common tools used in managed care are:[75]

- security within data processing systems, such as confidential passwords;
- authorized data entry procedures so that those who enter data cannot pay claims;
- system accountability so that those who maintain provider records do not pay claims; and
- limiting the dollar amounts payable to newly hired staff or contracted providers until a probationary period is completed.

One important method of controlling abuse is to maintain strict confidentiality of patient records. Medical claims and patient records contain highly sensitive information that should never be revealed to anyone inside or outside the organization who does not give direct patient services. Staff must be trained in procedures for maintaining confidentiality; generally, they are asked to sign a statement promising to maintain confidentiality of patient information. MIS may be used to assign confidentiality codes to certain patient records (e.g., claims for psychiatric care) to flag those records for assignment to a higher-level claims reviewer.

Externally, a managed care organization needs to be vigilant in controlling for fraud and abuse.[76] Outside providers need to be audited for inflated or inappropriate charges. "Red flags" or triggers can be used in such audits. For example, a flag can highlight illogical combinations of medical services (e.g., medical procedures performed on persons of the inappropriate gender).

Some common flags are:

- all hospital claims over a certain amount (e.g., $15,000);
- more than 50 percent of hospital charges for non-room-and-board services; and
- inappropriate service for diagnosis (e.g., not ordering certain laboratory tests for a diagnosis of diabetes).

In the case of pharmaceutical costs, both providers and patients may perpetrate fraud. Attempts to curb pharmaceutical fraud include:

- requirements to use generic drugs;
- "red flags" for dispensed prescriptions costing over a certain amount (e.g., $125); and
- "red flags" for vague notations.

Networked or interorganization MIS systems can be used to detect pharmaceutical fraud and abuse. These systems often serve to discover abuse that can occur by incorrectly dispensing prescriptions. Cautions and checks are needed in all pharmaceutical systems to prevent dispensing incorrect drugs or dosages. Retrospectively, system checks can occur to compare physicians' orders with actual drugs and dosages dispensed.

MIS has been extremely useful in drug benefit programs in other ways. Current, sophisticated network systems are able to:

- check the eligibility of individuals seeking prescriptions;
- confirm whether prescriptions are covered by the insurer's plan or are a part of a plan's formulary of acceptable pharmaceuticals;
- indicate previous authorizations for special drug dispensing;
- validate whether quantities or dosages are within norms of generally accepted medical practice; and
- profile consumer information to prevent drug interactions, drug-to-disease interactions, or overuse of certain drugs (e.g., by flagging that a prescription may have been filled too soon).

The complexity of fraud and abuse detection problems stems, in part, from the diversity of health care services and the dynamics of regional variations. The characteristics of fraud-related activities can vary by type of health industry services (laboratory, physician, chiropractor, pharmacist), by organization (individual, clinic, institution), and by geography. This means that the characteristics of fraudulent behavior for a specialist in Missouri can be different from those for a specialist in New York. In addition, these characteristics can change over time.

To reduce the risk of fraud in electronic environments, the following actions can be taken:

- establishment of quality criteria for provider eligibility to participate in MIS systems or networks;

- application of certain contractual agreements governing medical and claims records with participating providers;

- development and use of a unique provider identification mechanism through which claims submitted electronically may be traced to their source;

- triggers or "red flags" that highlight unusual or suspicious activity for further review;

- flexibility to add new "red flags" in the electronic system as they are identified in statistical analyses;

- defining potential fraudulent activities or behaviors by health care specialty to identify high-risk suspects;

- historical tracking of overall behavior and individual components of behavior for providers over several years; and

- statistical analysis tools to define behavior patterns that are at high risk of being fraudulent.

If properly implemented, electronic data systems help detect health care fraud and abuse, increase quality, and reduce health care costs.

■ Data for Behavioral Health Measurement

Data development to assess cost and quality of behavioral health programs are an integral part of expanding access and service in this type of health care environment. For example, performance reports assist managed care organizations in contracting with or directing the services of behavioral health care staff. Such reports can include utilization data, clinical outcomes, and patient satisfaction surveys.

In managed behavioral health, care must be taken to control both overuse and underuse of services. Without controls, managed care, particularly capitated payment programs, can influence behavioral health providers to provide fewer services than are adequate. Computerized clinical information systems are being developed that emphasize selective case management in those cases where services require closer attention. Not all cases necessitate the costs and time of case management controls, yet selective cases do warrant such benefits in the interest of providing quality services.

In addition, behavioral health practitioners are being asked by managed care organizations to document the value of behavioral health services, to demonstrate appropriateness of care, and to confirm adequacy of resources to provide the services that are needed.

■ Data for Outcome Measures

As seen in Chapter 7, there is growing interest in examining outcome measures for improving quality and lowering health care costs. In order to use outcome measures effectively, data must be gathered in an accurate and effective manner. Data for outcome measures should be:

- collected on a large number of individuals, since a few cases may not give accurate or representative data;

- collected in a uniform manner and at the same point in diagnosis or treatment;

- risk-adjusted to account for the effects of such things as age, severity of illness, and risk factors for disease;

- risk-adjusted when comparing actual performance with predicted performance by calculating on the basis of averages for special groups; and

- calculated with statistical probability formulas in order to avoid conclusions based on chance.

■ Data Requirements of Certifying or Accrediting Organizations

Managed care organizations sometimes need to seek certification or accreditation from various outside, independent organizations to demonstrate accountability to external customers, to avoid burdensome state-specific regulation that can be waived if other accreditation is obtained, and to validate quality services. A number of organizations perform various certifying or accreditation activities for managed care organizations. Two major organizations are the Joint Commission on Accreditation of Healthcare Organizations (JCAHO) and the National Committee on Quality Assurance (NCQA).

The Joint Commission on Accreditation of Healthcare Organizations (JCAHO)

The JCAHO is a private, voluntary organization that has a major impact on health care organizations in the United States. It began surveying hospitals in 1918, and what began as an accrediting organization setting minimal standards for hospitals has grown to an organization that accredits all types of health care organizations. Emphasis has moved along a continuum from minimal standards to medical audits to problem-oriented studies to ongoing monitoring of departmental standards to organizationwide continuous quality performance.

To ascertain accreditation, the JCAHO sends survey teams to health care organizations to gather data related to:

- organizationwide quality improvement and leadership in CQI;
- external and internal customer needs and satisfaction;
- work processes of management and various disciplines; and
- financial stability.

A JCAHO survey and accreditation process examines all elements of a health care organization by using explicit standards. An organization's MIS is one area that is evaluated. The standards for MIS evaluation include requirements that a health care organization identify its internal and external information needs, design a system that is appropriate, and capture and use accurate data.

All areas of a JCAHO assessment are measured by dimensions of performance. These include:

- efficiency,
- appropriateness,
- availability,
- timeliness,
- continuity,
- safety, and
- respect and caring.

A goal of the JCAHO is to encourage health care organizations to develop a continuous cycle for improving performance. Each organization should have an internal database of information that can be compared to similar information from outside the organization. Assessment should be conducted to determine if improvement is needed. Organizations are encouraged to use a process similar to FOCUS-PDCA for process improvement and performance-focused accreditation.

For health care organizations that wish to have or need JCAHO accreditation, the CQI model is becoming the standard of the industry. For those who do not wish to have such accreditation, the JCAHO Manuals of Accreditation are excellent guideposts for collecting useful data and developing new processes for improving quality and effectiveness.

The JCAHO has now directed its focus to outcome, process, and excellence in care. This new focus has lead the JCAHO into the area of indicator development for hospitals to create standards of care.

The indicator measurement system (IMSystem) develops "flags" that indicate areas for more detailed analysis. Variance in expected rates may indicate that there is a problem. Data used for the IMSystem include sentinel events which are always triggers for further analysis or review. Data for the IMSystem also are derived from aggregate data of persons, processes, and frequency levels. A thorough process of testing indicator validity and reliability is now taking place at participating JCAHO-accredited hospitals, with ten areas being put into a voluntary survey process by 1995. Hospitals participating in the IMSystem provide required data elements to the JCHAO, which assesses and processes this information.

The IMSystem data elements and requirements for automated data collection aim to:

- collect reliable and accurate data;
- generate reports that identify missing data;
- accurately calculate indicator categories for each episode of care;
- generate reports to assist in interpreting and using indicator data; and
- prepare and create data files in a proper format.

Development of the IMSystem is expected to eventually result in "report cards." The JCHAO reports quarterly to all who participate in the indicator project. These reports show a hospital's performance compared to that of other participants for each indicator. In the future, the JCAHO expects to provide other types of comparative reports, such as by region or hospital type, that will be available to payers, employers, patients, and other interested parties. Some health care network systems and regional medical organizations currently use report cards about clinical practice, outcome measures, or other data to allow payers and potential patients to compare cost and efficacy of health care.

The National Committee on Quality Assurance

The National Committee on Quality Assurance (NCQA), established in 1979, accredits prepaid managed care organizations and HMOs of all types. The NCQA uses review teams to gather data and assess quality, credentialing, utilization management, customer rights, preventive health services, and medical records.

In addition to the review and accreditation process for HMOs and managed care organizations, the NCQA has developed a core set of performance measures called Health Plan Employer Data and Information Set (HEDIS) 2.0. HEDIS was developed to serve the employer as purchaser of managed care but it can be adapted to serve the needs of other purchasers.

HEDIS 2.0 was developed in response to a need to let health care plans and employers "more accurately evaluate and trend health plan performance and, as the measures are refined, to use them in a comparative manner."[77] Five major areas of performance are measured in HEDIS 2.0. They are quality, access and patient satisfaction, membership and utilization, finance, and descriptive information on the health plan. The criteria for data in each area are that they: 1) be relevant to the employer community; 2) be reasonable for health plans to develop and provide; and 3) have potential impact on improving the process of care delivery.

NCQA is also developing a "report card" system from HEDIS 2.0 information for purchasers and consumers to learn if a plan is providing the most value for their health care dollar. The "report card" also seeks to make providers accountable for their performance.

To participate in the "report card" process, plans must conduct an internal audit of their information capabilities to demonstrate that they:

- can quickly enter data into the plan's administrative database;
- have access to previous years' data;
- capture data from patient encounter forms and diagnosis data;
- accurately code data; and
- carefully account for all costs in data.

The demands of accountability and "report cards" in managed care clearly require sophisticated MIS systems to accurately capture clinical, management, and financial data.

■ Summary

Data collection and data collection systems are essential components of any type of health care organization, especially for managed health care plans. Managed health care plans are complex organizations with competing demands for quality, cost and utilization control, and payer and customer satisfaction. The collection of accurate, timely, and relevant data is central to managing high-quality, cost-effective, and solvent managed care plans. The types of data needed are those that help define technical quality, acceptability of services to payers and patients, comparability to competing organizations and plans, and accessibility to services.

■ Key Terms

Administrative files
Administrative systems
Applications reporting
   systems
Appropriateness of
   care
Audits
Automated services
Behavioral health
Capitated payment
   arrangements
Capitation rates
Claims adjudication
Clinical managers
Clinical outcomes
Clinical systems
Coding
Comparative practice
   patterns
Confidentiality
Confidentiality codes
Cost analysis
Cost per member per
   month ($PMPM)
Credentialing
Cumulative member
   months (CMMs)
Customer satisfaction
Customer service
   representatives
Database forecasting
Database management
   systems

Decision support
   systems (DSS)
Demand analysis
Formulary
Fraud and abuse
Frequency
Gross Margin PMPM
Health Care Financing
   Administration
   (HCFA)
Health Plan Employer
   Data and Information
   Set (HEDIS) 2.0
Hospital days per 1,000
Hospital expense PMPM
Hospital readmission
   rates
Incurred but not
   reported claims
   (IBNR)
Indicators
Inputs
Insurance claims data
Joint Commission on
   Accreditation of
   Healthcare
   Organizations
   (JCAHO)
Laboratory reports
Litigation
Management
   Information Systems
   (MIS)

Medical records
National Committee on
   Quality Assurance
   (NCQA)
Networks systems
Other expenses PMPM
Outpatient forecasting
Outputs
Passwords
Patient satisfaction
   surveys
Peer review committees
Performance reports
Per member per month
   (PMPM)
Per member per year
   (PMPY)
Physician expense
   PMPM
Process
Productivity reports
Profiling
Profit margin
Prospective
Quality assurance
   committees
Quality improvement
   teams
Rates
"Red flags"
Regional medical
   organizations
"Report cards"

Retrospective	Sentinel events	Underutilization
Risk-adjusted	Systems modeling	Utilization control
Risk factors	Treatment practice	Utilization rates
Selective case management	Triggers	Variation

Appendix A

HEALTH MAINTENANCE ORGANIZATION ACT OF 1973

Table of Contents

Section 1. Short title and table of contents.
Section 2. Health maintenance organizations.

          "TITLE XIII—HEALTH MAINTENANCE ORGANIZATIONS

"Sec. 1301. Requirements for health maintenance organizations.
"Sec. 1302. Definitions.
"Sec. 1303. Grants and contracts for feasibility surveys.
"Sec. 1304. Grants, contracts, and loan guarantees for planning and for initial development costs.
"Sec. 1305. Loans and loan guarantees for initial operation costs.
"Sec. 1306. Application requirements.
"Sec. 1307. Administration of assistance programs.
"Sec. 1308. General provisions relating to loan guarantees and loans.
"Sec. 1309. Authorizations of appropriations.
"Sec. 1310. Employees' health benefits plans.
"Sec. 1311. Restrictive State laws and practices.
"Sec. 1312. Continued regulation of health maintenance organizations.
"Sec. 1313. Limitation on source of funding for health maintenance organizations.
"Sec. 1314. Program evaluation.
"Sec. 1315. Annual report.".
Section 3. Quality assurance.
Section 4. Health care quality assurance programs study.
Section 5. Reports respecting medically underserved areas and population groups and non-metropolitan areas.
Section 6. Health services for Indians and domestic agricultural migratory and seasonal workers.
Section 7. Conforming amendments.

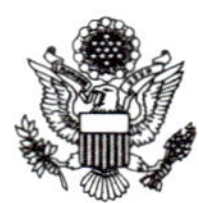

Public Law 93-222
93rd Congress, S. 14
December 29, 1973

An Act

87 STAT. 914

To amend the Public Health Service Act to provide assistance and encouragement for the establishment and expansion of health maintenance organizations,
and for other purposes.

*Be it enacted by the Senate and House of Representatives of the
United States of America in Congress assembled,*

Health Mainte-
nance Organiza-
tion Act of
1973.

SHORT TITLE AND TABLE OF CONTENTS

SECTION 1. This Act, with the following table of contents, may be
cited as the "Health Maintenance Organization Act of 1973".

TABLE OF CONTENTS

Sec. 1. Short title and table of contents.
Sec. 2. Health maintenance organizations.

"TITLE XIII—HEALTH MAINTENANCE ORGANIZATIONS

"Sec. 1301. Requirements for health maintenance organizations.
"Sec. 1302. Definitions.
"Sec. 1303. Grants and contracts for feasibility surveys.
"Sec. 1304. Grants, contracts, and loan guarantees for planning and for
            initial development costs.
"Sec. 1305. Loans and loan guarantees for initial operation costs.
"Sec. 1306. Application requirements.
"Sec. 1307. Administration of assistance programs.
"Sec. 1308. General provisions relating to loan guarantees and loans.
"Sec. 1309. Authorizations of appropriations.
"Sec. 1310. Employees' health benefits plans.
"Sec. 1311. Restrictive State laws and practices.
"Sec. 1312. Continued regulation of health maintenance organizations.
"Sec. 1313. Limitation on source of funding for health maintenance orga-
            nizations.
"Sec. 1314. Program evaluation.
"Sec. 1315. Annual report.".
Sec. 3. Quality assurance.
Sec. 4. Health care quality assurance programs study.
Sec. 5. Reports respecting medically underserved areas and population groups
        and non-metropolitan areas.
Sec. 6. Health services for Indians and domestic agricultural migratory and
        seasonal workers.
Sec. 7. Conforming amendments.

HEALTH MAINTENANCE ORGANIZATIONS

SEC. 2. The Public Health Service Act is amended by adding after
title XII the following new title:

Ante, p. 594.

"TITLE XIII—HEALTH MAINTENANCE ORGANIZATIONS

"REQUIREMENTS FOR HEALTH MAINTENANCE ORGANIZATIONS

"SEC. 1301. (a) For purposes of this title, the term 'health maintenance organization' means a legal entity which (1) provides basic and
supplemental health services to its members in the manner prescribed
by subsection (b), and (2) is organized and operated in the manner
prescribed by subsection (c).

Definition.

99-081 O

87 STAT. 915

Basic health
services.

"(b) A health maintenance organization shall provide, without limitations as to time or cost other than those prescribed by or under this title, basic and supplemental health services to its members in the following manner:

"(1) Each member is to be provided basic health services for a basic health services payment which (A) is to be paid on a periodic basis without regard to the dates health services (within the basic health services) are provided; (B) is fixed without regard to the frequency, extent, or kind of health service (within the basic health services) actually furnished; (C) is fixed under a community rating system; and (D) may be supplemented by additional nominal payments which may be required for the provision of specific services (within the basic health services), except that such payments may not be required where or in such a manner that they serve (as determined under regulations of the Secretary) as a barrier to the delivery of health services. Such additional nominal payments shall be fixed in accordance with the regulations of the Secretary.

"(2) For such payment or payments (hereinafter in this title referred to as 'supplemental health services payments') as the health maintenance organization may require in addition to the basic health services payment, the organization shall provide to each of its members each health service (A) which is included in supplemental health services (as defined in section 1302(2)), (B) for which the required health manpower are available in the area served by the organization, and (C) for the provision of which the member has contracted with the organization. Supplemental health services payments which are fixed on a prepayment basis shall be fixed under a community rating system.

"(3) The services of health professionals which are provided as basic health services shall be provided through health professionals who are members of the staff of the health maintenance organization or through a medical group (or groups) or individual practice association (or associations), except that this paragraph shall not apply in the case of (A) health professionals' services which the organization determines, in conformity with regulations of the Secretary, are unusual or infrequently used, or (B) any basic health service provided a member of the health maintenance organization other than by such a health professional because it was medically necessary that the service be provided to the member before he could have it provided by such a health professional. For purposes of this paragraph, the term 'health professionals' means physicians, dentists, nurses, podiatrists, optometrists, and such other individuals engaged in the delivery of health services as the Secretary may by regulation designate.

"Health
professionals."

"(4) Basic health services (and supplemental health services in the case of the members who have contracted therefor) shall within the area served by the health maintenance organization be available and accessible to each of its members promptly as appropriate and in a manner which assures continuity, and when medically necessary be available and accessible twenty-four hours a day and seven days a week. A member of a health maintenance organization shall be reimbursed by the organization for his expenses in securing basic or supplemental health services other than through the organization if it was medically necessary that the services be provided before he could secure them through the organization.

87 STAT. 916

"(c) Each health maintenance organization shall—

"(1) have a fiscally sound operation and adequate provision against the risk of insolvency which is satisfactory to the Secretary;

"(2) assume full financial risk on a prospective basis for the provision of basic health services, except that a health maintenance organization may obtain insurance or make other arrangements (A) for the cost of providing to any member basic health services the aggregate value of which exceeds $5,000 in any year, (B) for the cost of basic health services provided to its members other than through the organization because medical necessity required their provision before they could be secured through the organization, and (C) for not more than 90 per centum of the amount by which its costs for any of its fiscal years exceed 115 per centum of its income for such fiscal year;

"(3) enroll persons who are broadly representative of the various age, social, and income groups within the area it serves, except that in the case of a health maintenance organization which has a medically underserved population located (in whole or in part) in the area it serves, not more than 75 per centum of the members of that organization may be enrolled from the medically underserved population unless the area in which such population resides is also a rural area (as designated by the Secretary);

"(4) have an open enrollment period of not less than thirty days at least once during each consecutive twelve-month period during which enrollment period it accepts, up to its capacity, individuals in the order in which they apply for enrollment, except that if the organization demonstrates to the satisfaction of the Secretary that—

"(A) it has enrolled, or will be compelled to enroll, a disproportionate number of individuals who are likely to utilize its services more often than an actuarially determined average (as determined under regulations of the Secretary) and enrollment during an open enrollment period of an additional number of such individuals will jeopardize its economic viability, or

"(B) if it maintained an open enrollment period it would not be able to comply with the requirements of paragraph (3),

the Secretary may waive compliance by the organization with the open enrollment requirement of this paragraph for not more than three consecutive twelve-month periods and may provide additional waivers to that organization if it makes the demonstration required by subparagraph (A) or (B);

"(5) not expel or refuse to re-enroll any member because of his health status or his requirements for health services;

"(6) be organized in such a manner that assures that (A) at least one-third of the membership of the policymaking body of the health maintenance organization will be members of the organization, and (B) there will be equitable representation on such body of members from medically underserved populations served by the organization;

"(7) be organized in such a manner that provides meaningful procedures for hearing and resolving grievances between the health maintenance organization (including the medical group or groups and other health delivery entities providing health services for the organization) and the members of the organization;

"(8) have organizational arrangements, established in accordance with regulations of the Secretary, for an ongoing quality assurance program for its health services which program (A) stresses health outcomes, and (B) provides review by physicians

- 4 -

and other health professionals of the process followed in the provision of health services;

"(9) provide medical social services for its members and encourage and actively provide for its members health education services, education in the appropriate use of health services, and education in the contribution each member can make to the maintenance of his own health;

"(10) provide, or make arrangements for, continuing education for its health professional staff; and

"(11) provide, in accordance with regulations of the Secretary (including safeguards concerning the confidentiality of the doctor-patient relationship), an effective procedure for developing, compiling, evaluating, and reporting to the Secretary, statistics and other information (which the Secretary shall publish and disseminate on an annual basis and which the health maintenance organization shall disclose, in a manner acceptable to the Secretary, to its members and the general public) relating to (A) the cost of its operations, (B) the patterns of utilization of its services, (C) the availability, accessibility, and acceptability of its services, (D) to the extent practical, developments in the health status of its members, and (E) such other matters as the Secretary may require.

"DEFINITIONS

"Sec. 1302. For purposes of this title:
"(1) The term 'basic health services' means—
"(A) physician services (including consultant and referral services by a physician);
"(B) inpatient and outpatient hospital services;
"(C) medically necessary emergency health services;
"(D) short-term (not to exceed twenty visits), outpatient evaluative and crisis intervention mental health services;
"(E) medical treatment and referral services (including referral services to appropriate ancillary services) for the abuse of or addiction to alcohol and drugs;
"(F) diagnostic laboratory and diagnostic and therapeutic radiologic services;
"(G) home health services; and
"(H) preventive health services (including voluntary family planning services, infertility services, preventive dental care for children, and children's eye examinations conducted to determine the need for vision correction).

If a service of a physician described in the preceding sentence may also be provided under applicable State law by a dentist, optometrist, or podiatrist, a health maintenance organization may provide such service through a dentist, optometrist, or podiatrist (as the case may be) licensed to provide such service. For purposes of this paragraph, the term 'home health services' means health services provided at a member's home by health care personnel, as prescribed or directed by the responsible physician or other authority designated by the health maintenance organization. A health maintenance organization is authorized, in connection with the prescription of drugs, to maintain, review, and evaluate (in accordance with regulations of the Secretary) a drug use profile of its members receiving such service, evaluate patterns of drug utilization to assure optimum drug therapy, and provide for instruction of its members and of health professionals in the use of prescription and non-prescription drugs.

"(2) The term 'supplemental health services' means—
"(A) services of facilities for intermediate and long-term care;

87 STAT. 918

"(B) vision care not included as a basic health service under paragraph (1)(A) or (1)(H);

"(C) dental services not included as a basic health service under paragraph (1)(A) or (1)(H);

"(D) mental health services not included as a basic health service under paragraph (1)(D);

"(E) long-term physical medicine and rehabilitative services (including physical therapy); and

"(F) the provision of prescription drugs prescribed in the course of the provision by the health maintenance organization of a basic health service or a service described in the preceding subparagraphs of this paragraph.

If a service of a physician described in the preceding sentence may also be provided under applicable State law by a dentist, optometrist, or podiatrist, a health maintenance organization may provide such service through an optometrist, dentist, or podiatrist (as the case may be) licensed to provide such service. A health maintenance organization is authorized, in connection with the prescription or provision of prescription drugs, to maintain, review, and evaluate (in accordance with regulations of the Secretary) a drug use profile of its members receiving such services, evaluate patterns of drug utilization to assure optimum drug therapy, and provide for instruction of its members and of health professionals in the use of prescription and non-prescription drugs.

"(3) The term 'member' when used in connection with a health maintenance organization means an individual who has entered into a contractual arrangement, or on whose behalf a contractual arrangement has been entered into, with the organization under which the organization assumes the responsibility for the provision to such individual of basic health services and of such supplemental health services as may be contracted for.

"(4) The term 'medical group' means a partnership, association, or other group—

"(A) which is composed of health professionals licensed to practice medicine or osteopathy and of such other licensed health professionals (including dentists, optometrists, and podiatrists) as are necessary for the provision of health services for which the group is responsible;

"(B) a majority of the members of which are licensed to practice medicine or osteopathy; and

"(C) the members of which (i) as their principal professional activity and as a group responsibility engage in the coordinated practice of their profession for a health maintenance organization; (ii) pool their income from practice as members of the group and distribute it among themselves according to a prearranged salary or drawing account or other plan; (iii) share medical and other records and substantial portions of major equipment and of professional, technical, and administrative staff; (iv) utilize such additional professional personnel, allied health professions personnel, and other health personnel (as specified in regulations of the Secretary) as are available and appropriate for the effective and efficient delivery of the services of the members of the group; and (v) arrange for and encourage continuing education in the field of clinical medicine and related areas for the members of the group.

"(5) The term 'individual practice association' means a partnership, corporation, association, or other legal entity which has entered into a services arrangement (or arrangements) with persons who are licensed to practice medicine, osteopathy, dentistry, podiatry, optome-

87 STAT. 919

try, or other health profession in a State and a majority of whom are licensed to practice medicine or osteopathy. Such an arrangement shall provide—

"(A) that such persons shall provide their professional services in accordance with a compensation arrangement established by the entity; and

"(B) to the extent feasible (i) that such persons shall utilize such additional professional personnel, allied health professions personnel, and other health personnel (as specified in regulations of the Secretary) as are available and appropriate for the effective and efficient delivery of the services of the persons who are parties to the arrangement, (ii) for the sharing by such persons of medical and other records, equipment, and professional, technical, and administrative staff, and (iii) for the arrangement and encouragement of the continuing education of such persons in the field of clinical medicine and related areas.

"(6) The term 'section 314(a) State health planning agency' means the agency of a State which administers or supervises the administration of a State's health planning functions under a State plan approved under section 314(a) (hereinafter in this title referred to as a 'section 314(a) plan'); and the term 'section 314(b) areawide health planning agency' means a public or nonprofit private agency or organization which has developed a comprehensive regional, metropolitan, or other local area plan or plans referred to in section 314(b) (hereinafter in this title referred to as a 'section 314(b) plan').

80 Stat. 1181.
42 USC 246.

"(7) The term 'medically underserved population' means the population of an urban or rural area designated by the Secretary as an area with a shortage of personal health services or a population group designated by the Secretary as having a shortage of such services. Such a designation may be made by the Secretary only after consideration of the comments (if any) of (A) each section 314(a) State health planning agency whose section 314(a) plan covers (in whole or in part) such urban or rural area or the area in which such population group resides, and (B) each section 314(b) areawide health planning agency whose section 314(b) plan covers (in whole or in part) such urban or rural area or the area in which such population group resides.

"(8) The term 'community rating system' means a system of fixing rates of payments for health services. Under such a system rates of payments may be determined on a per-person or per-family basis and may vary with the number of persons in a family, but except as otherwise authorized in the next sentence, such rates must be equivalent for all individuals and for all families of similar composition. The following differentials in rates of payments may be established under such system:

"(A) Nominal differentials in such rates may be established to reflect the different administrative costs of collecting payments from the following categories of members:

"(i) Individual members (including their families).

"(ii) Small groups of members (as determined under regulations of the Secretary).

"(iii) Large groups of members (as determined under regulations of the Secretary).

"(B) Differentials in such rates may be established for members enrolled in a health maintenance organization pursuant to a contract with a governmental authority under section 1079 or 1086 of title 10, United States Code, or under any other governmental program (other than the health benefits program authorized by chapter 89 of title 5, United States Code) or any health

80 Stat. 863.

5 USC 8901.

87 STAT. 920

benefits program for employees of States, political subdivisions of States, and other public entities.

"(9) The term 'non-metropolitan area' means an area no part of which is within an area designated as a standard metropolitan statistical area by the Office of Management and Budget and which does not contain a city whose population exceeds fifty thousand individuals.

"GRANTS AND CONTRACTS FOR FEASIBILITY SURVEYS

"SEC. 1303. (a) The Secretary may make grants to and enter into contracts with public or nonprofit private entities for projects for surveys or other activities to determine the feasibility of developing and operating or expanding the operation of health maintenance organizations.

"(b) An application for a grant or contract under this section shall contain—

"(1) assurances satisfactory to the Secretary that, in conducting surveys or other activities with assistance under a grant or contract under this section, the applicant will (A) cooperate with the section 314(b) areawide health planning agency (if any) whose section 314(b) plan covers (in whole or in part) the area for which the survey or other activity will be conducted, and (B) notify the medical society serving such area of such surveys or other activities; and

80 Stat. 1181;
84 Stat. 1304.
42 USC 246.

"(2) such other information as the Secretary may by regulation prescribe.

"(c) In considering applications for grants and contracts under this section, the Secretary shall give priority to an application which contains or is supported by assurances satisfactory to the Secretary that at the time the health maintenance organization for which such application or proposal is submitted first becomes operational not less than 30 per centum of its members will be members of a medically underserved population.

"(d)(1) Except as provided in paragraph (2), the following limitations apply with respect to grants and contracts made under this section:

Limitations.

"(A) If a project has been assisted with a grant or contract under subsection (a), the Secretary may not make any other grant or enter into any other contract under this section for such project.

"(B) Any project for which a grant is made or contract entered into must be completed within twelve months from the date the grant is made or contract entered into.

"(2) The Secretary may make not more than one additional grant or enter into not more than one additional contract for a project for which a grant has previously been made or a contract previously entered into, and he may permit additional time (up to twelve months) for completion of the project if he determines that the additional grant or contract (as the case may be), or additional time, or both, is needed to adequately complete the project.

"(e) The amount to be paid by the United States under a grant made, or contract entered into, under subsection (a) shall be determined by the Secretary, except that (1) the amount to be paid by the United States under any single grant or contract for any project may not exceed $50,000, and (2) the aggregate of the amounts to be paid by the United States for any project under such subsection under grants or contracts, or both, may not exceed the greater of (A) 90 per centum of the cost of such project (as determined under regulations of the Secretary), or (B) in the case of a project for a health maintenance organization which will serve a medically underserved

87 STAT. 921

population, such greater percentage (up to 100 per centum) of such cost as the Secretary may prescribe if he determines that the ceiling on the grants and contracts for such project should be determined by such greater percentage.

"(f) Payments under grants under this section may be made in advance or by way of reimbursement and at such intervals and on such conditions as the Secretary finds necessary.

"(g) Contracts may be entered into under this section without regard to sections 3648 and 3709 of the Revised Statutes (31 U.S.C. 529; 41 U.S.C. 5).

Post, p.930.

"(h) Payments under grants and contracts under this section shall be made from appropriations made under section 1309(a).

"(i) Of the sums appropriated for any fiscal year under section 1309(a) for grants and contracts under this section, not less than 20 per centum shall be set aside and obligated in such fiscal year for projects (1) to determine the feasibility of developing and operating or expanding the operation of health maintenance organizations which the Secretary determines may reasonably be expected to have after their development or expansion not less than 66 per centum of their membership drawn from residents of non-metropolitan areas, and (2) the applications for which meet the requirements of this title for approval. Sums set aside in the fiscal year ending June 30, 1974, or June 30, 1975, for projects described in the preceding sentence but not obligated in such fiscal year for grants and contracts under this section because of a lack of applicants for projects meeting the requirements of such sentence shall remain available for obligation under this section in the succeeding fiscal year for projects other than those described in clause (1) of such sentence.

"GRANTS, CONTRACTS, AND LOAN GUARANTEES FOR PLANNING AND FOR INITIAL DEVELOPMENT COSTS

"SEC. 1304. (a) The Secretary may—

"(1) make grants to and enter into contracts with public or nonprofit private entities for planning projects for the establishment of health maintenance organizations or for the significant expansion of the membership of, or areas served by, health maintenance organizations; and

"(2) guarantee to non-Federal lenders payment of the principal of and the interest on loans made to private entities (other than nonprofit private entities) for planning projects for the establishment or expansion of health maintenance organizations to serve medically underserved populations.

Planning projects assisted under this subsection shall include development of plans for the marketing of the services of the health maintenance organization.

"(b)(1) The Secretary may— ,

"(A) make grants to and enter into contracts with public or nonprofit private entities for projects for the initial development of health maintenance organizations; and

"(B) guarantee to non-Federal lenders payment of the principal of and the interest on loans made to any private entity (other than a nonprofit private entity) for a project for the initial development of a health maintenance organization which will serve a medically underserved population.

'Initial development."

"(2) For purposes of this section, the term 'initial development' when used to describe a project for which assistance is authorized by this subsection includes significant expansion of the membership of, or the area served by, a health maintenance organization. Funds under grants and contracts under this subsection and under loans guaranteed under this subsection may only be utilized for such purposes as the Secretary may prescribe in regulations. Such purposes may include (A) the implementation of an enrollment campaign for such an organization, (B) the detailed design of and arrangements for the health services to be provided by such an organization, (C) the development of administrative and internal organizational arrangements, including fiscal control and fund accounting procedures, and the development of a capital financing program, (D) the recruitment of personnel for such an organization and the conduct of training activities for such personnel, and (E) the payment of architects' and engineers' fees.

"(3) A grant or contract under this subsection may only be made or entered into for initial development costs in the one-year period beginning on the first day of the first month in which such grant or contract is made or entered into. The number of grants made for any initial development project under this subsection when added to the number of contracts entered into for such project under this subsection may not exceed three. A loan guarantee under this subsection may only be made for a loan (or loans) for such costs incurred in a period not to exceed three years.

"(c)(1) An application for a grant, contract, or loan guarantee under subsection (a) for a planning project shall contain assurances satisfactory to the Secretary that in carrying out the planning project for which the grant, contract, or loan guarantee is sought, the applicant will (A) cooperate with the section 314(b) areawide health planning agency (if any) whose section 314(b) plan covers (in whole or in part) the area proposed to be served by the health maintenance organization for which the planning project will be conducted, and (B) notify the medical society serving such area of the planning project.

80 Stat. 1181;
84 Stat. 1304.
42 USC 246.

"(2) If the Secretary makes a grant or loan guarantee or enters into a contract under subsection (a) for a planning project for a health maintenance organization, he may, within the period in which the planning project must be completed, make a grant or loan guarantee or enter into a contract under subsection (b) for the initial development of that health maintenance organization; but no grant or loan guarantee may be made or contract entered into under subsection (b) for initial development of a health maintenance organization unless the Secretary determines that (A) sufficient planning for its establishment or expansion (as the case may be) has been conducted by the applicant for the grant, contract, or loan guarantee, and (B) the feasibility of establishing and operating, or of expanding, the health maintenance organization has been established by the applicant.

"(d) In considering applications for grants and contracts under this section, the Secretary shall give priority to an application which contains or is supported by assurances satisfactory to the Secretary that at the time the health maintenance organization for which such application is submitted first becomes operational not less than 30 per centum of its members will be members of a medically underserved population.

"(e)(1) Except as provided in paragraph (2), the following limitations apply with respect to grants, loan guarantees, and contracts made under subsection (a) of this section:

Limitations.

"(A) If a planning project has been assisted with grant, loan guarantee, or contract under subsection (a), the Secretary may not make any other planning grant or loan guarantee or enter into any other planning contract for such project under this section.

"(B) Any project for which a grant or loan guarantee is made or contract entered into must be completed within twelve months

87 STAT. 923

from the date the grant or loan guarantee is made or contract entered into.

"(2) The Secretary may not make more than one additional grant or loan guarantee or enter into not more than one additional contract for a planning project for which a grant or loan guarantee has previously been made or a contract previously entered into, and he may permit additional time (up to twelve months) for completion of the project if he determines that the additional grant, loan guarantee, or contract (as the case may be), or additional time, or both, is needed to adequately complete the project.

"(f)(1) The amount to be paid by the United States under a grant made, or contract entered into, under subsection (a) for a planning project, and (except as provided in paragraph (3) of this subsection) the amount of principal of a loan for a planning project which may be guaranteed under such subsection, shall be determined by the Secretary, except that (A) the amount to be paid by the United States under any single grant or contract, and the amount of principal of any single loan guaranteed under such subsection, may not exceed $125,000, and (B) the aggregate of the amounts to be paid for any project by the United States under grants or contracts, or both, under such subsection, and the aggregate amount of principal of loans guaranteed under such subsection for any project, may not exceed the greater of (i) 90 per centum of the cost of such project (as determined under regulations of the Secretary), or (ii) in the case of a project for a health maintenance organization which will serve a medically underserved population, such greater percentage (up to 100 per centum) of such cost as the Secretary may prescribe if he determines that the ceiling on the grants, contracts, and loan guarantees (or any combination thereof) for such project should be determined by such greater percentage.

"(2) The amount to be paid by the United States under a grant made, or contract entered into, under subsection (b) for an initial development project, and (except as provided in paragraph (3) of this subsection) the amount of principal of a loan for an initial development project which may be guaranteed under such subsection, shall be determined by the Secretary; except that the amounts to be paid by the United States for any initial development project under grants or contracts, or both, under such subsection, and the aggregate amount of principal of loans guaranteed under such subsection for any project, may not exceed the lesser of—

"(A) $1,000,000, or

"(B) an amount equal to the greater of (i) 90 per centum of the cost of such project (as determined under regulations of the Secretary), or (ii) in the case of a project for a health maintenance organization which will serve a medically underserved population, such greater percentage (up to 100 per centum) of such cost as the Secretary may prescribe if he determines that the ceiling on the grants, contracts, and loan guarantees (or any combination thereof) for such project should be determined by such greater percentage.

"(3) The cumulative total of the principal of the loans outstanding at any time with respect to which guarantees have been issued under this section may not exceed such limitations as may be specified in appropriation Acts.

"(g) Payments under grants under this section may be made in advance or by way of reimbursement and at such intervals and on such conditions as the Secretary finds necessary.

"(h) Contracts may be entered into under this section without regard to sections 3648 and 3709 of the Revised Statutes (31 U.S.C. 529; 41 U.S.C. 5).

87 STAT. 924

"(i) Payments under grants and contracts under this section shall be made from appropriations under section 1309(a). Post, p. 930.

"(j) Loan guarantees under subsection (a)(2) for planning projects may be made through the fiscal year ending June 30, 1976; and loan guarantees under subsection (b)(1)(B) for initial development projects may be made through the fiscal year ending June 30, 1977.

"(k)(1) Of the sums appropriated for any fiscal year under section 1309(a) for grants and contracts under subsection (a) of this section, not less than 20 per centum shall be set aside and obligated in such fiscal year for projects (A) to plan the establishment or expansion of health maintenance organizations which the Secretary determines may reasonably be expected to have after their establishment or expansion not less than 66 per centum of their membership drawn from residents of non-metropolitan areas, and (B) the applications for which meet the requirements of this title for approval. Sums set aside in the fiscal year ending June 30, 1974, or June 30, 1975, for projects described in the preceding sentence but not obligated in such fiscal year for grants and contracts under subsection (a) of this section because of a lack of applicants for projects meeting the requirements of such sentence shall remain available for obligation under such subsection in the succeeding fiscal year for projects other than those described in clause(A) of such sentence.

"(2) Of the sums appropriated for any fiscal year under section 1309(a) for grants and contracts under subsection (b) of this section, not less than 20 per centum shall be set aside and obligated in such fiscal year for projects (A) for the initial development of health maintenance organizations which the Secretary determines may reasonably be expected to have after their initial development not less than 66 per centum of their membership drawn from residents of non-metropolitan areas, and (B) the applications for which meet the requirements of this title for approval. Sums set aside in the fiscal year ending June 30, 1974, or in either of the next two fiscal years for projects described in the preceding sentence but not obligated in such fiscal year for grants and contracts under subsection (b) of this section because of a lack of applicants for projects meeting the requirements of such sentence shall remain available for obligation under such subsection in the succeeding fiscal year for projects other than those described in clause (A) of such sentence.

"LOANS AND LOAN GUARANTEES FOR INITIAL OPERATION COSTS

"SEC. 1305. (a) The Secretary may—

"(1) make loans to public or nonprofit private health maintenance organizations to assist them in meeting the amount by which their operating costs in the period of the first thirty-six months of their operation exceed their revenues in that period;

"(2) make loans to public or nonprofit private health maintenance organizations to assist them in meeting the amount by which their operating costs, which the Secretary determines are attributable to significant expansion in their membership or area served and which are incurred in the period of the first thirty-six months of their operation after such expansion, exceed their revenues in that period which the Secretary determines are attributable to such expansion; and

"(3) guarantee to non-Federal lenders payment of the principal of and the interest on loans made to any private health maintenance organization (other than a private nonprofit health maintenance organization) for the amounts referred to in paragraph (1) or (2), but only if such health maintenance organization will serve a medically underserved population. Non-Federal lenders, guaranteed payment, condition.

No loan or loan guarantee may be made under this subsection for the operating costs of a health maintenance organization unless the Secretary determines that the organization has made all reasonable attempts to meet such costs.

Limitations.

"(b)(1) Except as provided in paragraph (2), the principal amount of any loan made or guaranteed under subsection (a) in any fiscal year for a health maintenance organization may not exceed $1,000,000 and the aggregate amount of principal of loans made or guaranteed, or both, under this section for a health maintenance organization may not exceed $2,500,000.

"(2) The cumulative total of the principal of the loans outstanding at any time which have been directly made, or with respect to which guarantees have been issued, under subsection (a) may not exceed such limitations as may be specified in appropriation Acts.

Post, p. 930.

"(c) Loans under this section shall be made from the fund established under section 1308(e).

"(d) A loan or loan guarantee may be made under this section through the fiscal year ending June 30, 1978.

"(e) Of the sums used for loans under this section in any fiscal year from the loan fund established under section 1308(e), not less than 20 per centum shall be used for loans for projects (1) for the initial operation of health maintenance organizations which the Secretary determines have not less than 66 per centum of their membership drawn from residents of nonmetropolitan areas, and (2) the applications for which meet the requirements of this title for approval.

"APPLICATION REQUIREMENTS

"Sec. 1306. (a) No grant, contract, loan, or loan guarantee may be made under this title unless an application therefor has been submitted to, and approved by, the Secretary.

"(b) The Secretary may not approve an application for a grant, contract, loan, or loan guarantee under this title unless—

Ante, pp. 920, 921.

"(1) in the case of an application for assistance under section 1303 or 1304, such application meets the application requirements of such section and in the case of an application for a loan or loan guarantee, such application meets the requirements of section 1308;

"(2) he determines that the applicant making the application would not be able to complete the project or undertaking for which the application is submitted without the assistance applied for;

"(3) the application contains satisfactory specification of the existing or anticipated (A) population group or groups to be served by the proposed or existing health maintenance organization described in the application, (B) membership of such organization, (C) methods, terms, and periods of the enrollment of members of such organization, (D) estimated costs per member of the health and educational services to be provided by such organization and the nature of such costs, (E) sources of professional services for such organization, and organizational arrangements of such organization for providing health and educational services, (F) organizational arrangements of such organization for an ongoing quality assurance program in conformity with the

Ante, p. 914.

requirements of section 1301(c), (G) sources of prepayment and other forms of payment for the services to be provided by such organization, (H) facilities, and additional capital investments and sources of financing therefor, available to such organization to provide the level and scope of services proposed, (I) administrative, managerial, and financial arrangements and capabilities

87 STAT. 926

of such organization, (J) role for members in the planning and policymaking for such organization, (K) grievance procedures for members of such organization, and (L) evaluations of the support for and acceptance of such organization by the population to be served, the sources of operating support, and the professional groups to be involved or affected thereby;

"(4) contains or is supported by assurances satisfactory to the Secretary that the applicant making the application will, in accordance with such criteria as the Secretary shall by regulation prescribe, enroll, and maintain an enrollment of the maximum number of members that its available and potential resources (as determined under regulations of the Secretary) will enable it to effectively serve;

"(5) the section 314(b) areawide health planning agency whose section 314(b) plan covers (in whole or in part) the area to be served by the health maintenance organization for which such application is submitted, or if there is no such agency, the section 314(a) State health planning agency whose section 314(a) plan covers (in whole or in part) such area, has, in accordance with regulations of the Secretary under subsection (c) of this section, been provided an opportunity to review the application and to submit to the Secretary for his consideration its recommendations respecting approval of the application or if under applicable State law such an application may not be submitted without the approval of the section 314(b) areawide health planning agency or the section 314(a) State health planning agency, the required approval has been obtained;

80 Stat. 1181;
84 Stat. 1304.
42 USC 246.

"(6) in the case of an application made for a project which previously received a grant, contract, loan, or loan guarantee under this title, such application contains or is supported by assurances satisfactory to the Secretary that the applicant making the application has the financial capability to adequately carry out the purposes of such project and has developed and operated such project in accordance with the requirements of this title and with the plans contained in previous applications for such assistance; and

"(7) the application is submitted in such form and manner, and contains such additional information, as the Secretary shall prescribe in regulations.

An organization making multiple applications for more than one grant, contract, loan, or loan guarantee under this title, simultaneously or over the course of time, shall not be required to submit duplicate or redundant information but shall be required to update the specifications (required by paragraph (3)) respecting the existing or proposed health maintenance organization in such manner and with such frequency as the Secretary may by regulation prescribe.

Multiple applications.

"(c) The Secretary shall by regulation establish standards and procedures for section 314(b) areawide health planning agencies and section 314(a) State health planning agencies to follow in reviewing and commenting on applications for grants, contracts, loans, and loan guarantees under this title.

"ADMINISTRATION OF ASSISTANCE PROGRAMS

"SEC. 1307. (a)(1) Each recipient of a grant, contract, loan, or loan guarantee under this title shall keep such records as the Secretary shall prescribe, including records which fully disclose the amount and disposition by such recipient of the proceeds of the grant, contract, or

Record-
keeping.

87 STAT. 927

loan (directly made or guaranteed), the total cost of the undertaking in connection with which such assistance was given or used, the amount of that portion of the cost of the undertaking supplied by other sources, and such other records as will facilitate an effective audit.

"(2) The Secretary, or any of his duly authorized representatives, shall have access for the purpose of audit and examination to any books, documents, papers, and records of the recipients of a grant, contract, loan, or loan guarantee under this title which relate to such assistance.

Report to Secretary of H.E.W.

"(b) Upon expiration of the period for which a grant, contract, loan, or loan guarantee was provided an entity under this title, such entity shall make a full and complete report to the Secretary in such manner as he may by regulation prescribe. Each such report shall contain, among such other matters as the Secretary may by regulation require, descriptions of plans, developments, and operations relating to the matters referred to in section 1306(b)(3).

Ante, p. 925.

Post, p. 930.

"(c) If in any fiscal year the funds appropriated under section 1309 are insufficient to fund all applications approved under this title for that fiscal year, the Secretary shall, after applying the applicable priorities under sections 1303 and 1304, give priority to the funding of applications for projects which the Secretary determines are the most likely to be economically viable.

"(d) An entity which provides health services to a defined population on a prepaid basis and which has members who are entitled to insurance benefits under title XVIII of the Social Security Act or to medical assistance under a State plan approved under title XIX of such Act may be considered as a health maintenance organization for purposes of receiving assistance under this title if—

79 Stat. 291;
83 Stat. 1370.
42 USC 1395.
42 USC 1396.

"(1) with respect to its members who are entitled to such insurance benefits or to such medical assistance it (A) provides health services in accordance with section 1301(b), except that (i) it does not furnish to those members the health services (within the basic health services) for which it may not be compensated under such title XVIII or such State plan, and (ii) it does not fix the basic or supplemental health services payment for such members under a community rating system, and (B) is organized and operated in the manner prescribed by section 1301(c), except that it does not assume full financial risk on a prospective basis for the provision to such members of basic or supplemental health services with respect to which it is not required under such title XVIII or such State plan to assume such financial risk; and

"(2) with respect to its other members it provides health services in accordance with section 1301(b) and is organized and operated in the manner prescribed by section 1301(c).

"(e) In any fiscal year no loan guarantee may be made under this title if the making of such guarantee would cause the cumulative total of the principal of the loans guaranteed under this title in such fiscal year to exceed the amount of grant and contract funds obligated under this title in such fiscal year; except that this subsection shall not apply if the amount of grant and contract funds obligated under this title in such fiscal year equals the sums appropriated under section 1309 for grants and contracts for such fiscal year.

"GENERAL PROVISIONS RELATING TO LOAN GUARANTEES AND LOANS

"SEC. 1308. (a)(1) The Secretary may not approve an application for a loan guarantee under this title unless he determines that (A) the terms, conditions, security (if any), and schedule and amount of repayments with respect to the loan are sufficient to protect the finan-

87 STAT. 928

cial interests of the United States and are otherwise reasonable, including a determination that the rate of interest does not exceed such per centum per annum on the principal obligation outstanding as the Secretary determines to be reasonable, taking into account the range of interest rates prevailing in the private market for similar loans and the risks assumed by the United States, and (B) the loan would not be available on reasonable terms and conditions without the guarantee under this title.

"(2)(A) The United States shall be entitled to recover from the applicant for a loan guarantee under this title the amount of any payment made pursuant to such guarantee, unless the Secretary for good cause waives such right of recovery; and, upon making any such payment, the United States shall be subrogated to all of the rights of the recipient of the payments with respect to which the guarantee was made.

"(B) To the extent permitted by subparagraph (C), any terms and conditions applicable to a loan guarantee under this title (including terms and conditions imposed under subparagraph (D)) may be modified by the Secretary to the extent he determines it to be consistent with the financial interest of the United States.

"(C) Any loan guarantee made by the Secretary under this title shall be incontestable (i) in the hands of an applicant on whose behalf such guarantee is made unless the applicant engaged in fraud or misrepresentation in securing such guarantee, and (ii) as to any person (or his successor in interest) who makes or contracts to make a loan to such applicant in reliance thereon unless such person (or his successor in interest) engaged in fraud or misrepresentation in making or contracting to make such loan.

"(D) Guarantees of loans under this title shall be subject to such further terms and conditions as the Secretary determines to be necessary to assure that the purposes of this title will be achieved.

"(b)(1) The Secretary may not approve an application for a loan under this title unless— *Application requirements.*

"(A) the Secretary is reasonably satisfied that the applicant therefor will be able to make payments of principal and interest thereon when due, and

"(B) the applicant provides the Secretary with reasonable assurances that there will be available to it such additional funds as may be necessary to complete the project or undertaking with respect to which such loan is requested.

"(2) Any loan made under this title shall (A) have such security, (B) have such maturity date, (C) be repayable in such installments, (D) bear interest at a rate comparable to the current rate of interest prevailing, on the date the loan is made, with respect to loans guaranteed under this title, and (E) be subject to such other terms and conditions (including provisions for recovery in case of default), as the Secretary determines to be necessary to carry out the purposes of this title while adequately protecting the financial interests of the United States.

"(3) The Secretary may, for good cause but with due regard to the financial interests of the United States, waive any right of recovery which he has by reason of the failure of a borrower to make payments of principal of and interest on a loan made under this title, except that if such loan is sold and guaranteed, any such waiver shall have no effect upon the Secretary's guarantee of timely payment of principal and interest. *Right of recovery, waiver.*

"(c)(1) The Secretary may from time to time, but with due regard to the financial interests of the United States, sell loans made by him under this title. *Sale of loans.*

"(2) The Secretary may agree, prior to his sale of any such loan, to guarantee to the purchaser (and any successor in interest of the purchaser) compliance by the borrower with the terms and conditions of such loan. Any such agreement shall contain such terms and conditions as the Secretary considers necessary to protect the financial interests of the United States or as otherwise appropriate. Any such agreement may (A) provide that the Secretary shall act as agent of any such purchaser for the purpose of collecting from the borrower to which such loan was made and paying over to such purchaser, any payments of principal and interest payable by such organization under such loan; and (B) provide for the repurchase by the Secretary of any such loan on such terms and conditions as may be specified in the agreement. The full faith and credit of the United States is pledged to the payment of all amounts which may be required to be paid under any guarantee under this paragraph.

"(3) After any loan under this title to a public health maintenance organization has been sold and guaranteed under this subsection, interest paid on such loan which is received by the purchaser thereof (or his successor in interest) shall be included in the gross income of the purchaser of the loan (or his successor in interest) for the purpose of chapter 1 of the Internal Revenue Code of 1954.

"(4) Amounts received by the Secretary as proceeds from the sale of loans under this subsection shall be deposited in the loan fund established under subsection (e).

"(d)(1) There is established in the Treasury a loan guarantee fund (hereinafter in this subsection referred to as the 'fund') which shall be available to the Secretary without fiscal year limitation, in such amounts as may be specified from time to time in appropriation Acts, to enable him to discharge his responsibilities under loan guarantees issued by him under this title. There are authorized to be appropriated from time to time such amounts as may be necessary to provide the sums required for the fund. To the extent authorized in appropriation Acts, there shall also be deposited in the fund amounts received by the Secretary in connection with loan guarantees under this title and other property or assets derived by him from his operations respecting such loan guarantees, including any money derived from the sale of assets.

"(2) If at any time the sums in the funds are insufficient to enable the Secretary to discharge his responsibilities under guarantees issued by him under this title, he is authorized to issue to the Secretary of the Treasury notes or other obligations in such forms and denominations, bearing such maturities, and subject to such terms and conditions, as may be prescribed by the Secretary with the approval of the Secretary of the Treasury. Such notes or other obligations shall bear interest at a rate determined by the Secretary of the Treasury, taking into consideration the current average market yield on outstanding marketable obligations of the United States of comparable maturities during the month preceding the issuance of the notes or other obligations. The Secretary of the Treasury shall purchase any notes and other obligations issued under this paragraph and for that purpose he may use as a public debt transaction the proceeds from the sale of any securities issued under the Second Liberty Bond Act, and the purposes for which the securities may be issued under that Act are extended to include any purchase of such notes and obligations. The Secretary of the Treasury may at any time sell any of the notes or other obligations acquired by him under this paragraph. All redemptions, purchases, and sales by the Secretary of the Treasury of such notes or other obligations shall be treated as public debt transactions of the United States. Sums borrowed under this paragraph shall be deposited in the fund

87 STAT. 930

and redemption of such notes and obligations shall be made by the Secretary from the fund.

"(e) There is established in the Treasury a loan fund (hereinafter in this subsection referred to as the 'fund') which shall be available to the Secretary without fiscal year limitation, in such amounts as may be specified from time to time in appropriation Acts, to enable him to make loans under this title. There shall also be deposited in the fund amounts received by the Secretary as interest payments and repayment of principal on loans made under this title and other property or assets derived by him from his operations respecting such loans, from the sale of loans under subsection (c) of this section, or from the sale of assets.

"AUTHORIZATIONS OF APPROPRIATIONS

"SEC. 1309. (a) For the purpose of making payments under grants and contracts under sections 1303, 1304(a), and 1304(b), there are authorized to be appropriated $25,000,000 for the fiscal year ending June 30, 1974, $55,000,000 for the fiscal year ending June 30, 1975, and $85,000,000 for the fiscal year ending June 30, 1976; and for the purpose of making payments under grants and contracts under section 1304(b) for the fiscal year ending June 30, 1977, there is authorized to be appropriated $85,000,000.

"(b) There is authorized to be appropriated to the loan fund established under section 1308(e) $75,000,000 in the aggregrate for the fiscal years ending June 30, 1974, and June 30, 1975.

"EMPLOYEES' HEALTH BENEFITS PLANS

"SEC. 1310. (a) Each employer which is required during any calendar quarter to pay its employees the minimum wage specified by section 6 of the Fair Labor Standards Act of 1938 (or would be required to pay his employees such wage but for section 13(a) of such Act), and which during such calendar quarter employed an average number of employees of not less than twenty-five, shall, in accordance with regulations which the Secretary shall prescribe, include in any health benefits plan offered to its employees in the calendar year beginning after such calendar quarter the option of membership in qualified health maintenance organizations which are engaged in the provision of basic and supplemental health services in the areas in which such employees reside.

"(b) If there is more than one qualified health maintenance organization which is engaged in the provision of basic and supplemental health services in the area in which the employees of an employer subject to subsection (a) reside and if—

"(1) one or more of such organizations provides basic health services through professionals who are members of the staff of the organization or a medical group (or groups), and

"(2) one or more of such organizations provides such services through an individual practice association (or associations),

then of the qualified health maintenance organizations included in a health benefits plan of such employer pursuant to subsection (a) at least one shall be an organization which provides basic health services as described in clause (1) and at least one shall be an organization which provides basic health services as described in clause (2).

"(c) No employer shall be required to pay more for health benefits as a result of the application of this section than would otherwise be required by any prevailing collective bargaining agreement or other legally enforceable contract for the provision of health benefits between the employer and its employees. Failure of any employer to

87 STAT. 931

52 Stat. 1068;
63 Stat. 919.
29 USC 215.
"Qualified
health
maintenance
organization."

comply with the requirements of subsection (a) shall be considered a willful violation of section 15 of the Fair Labor Standards Act of 1938.

"(d) For purposes of this section, the term 'qualified health maintenance organization' means (1) a health maintenance organization which has provided assurances satisfactory to the Secretary that it provides basic and supplemental health services to its members in the manner prescribed by section 1301(b) and that it is organized and operated in the manner prescribed by section 1301(c), and (2) an entity which proposes to become a health maintenance organization and which the Secretary determines will when it becomes operational provide basic and supplemental health services to its members in the manner prescribed by section 1301(b) and will be organized and operated in the manner prescribed by section 1301(c).

"RESTRICTIVE STATE LAWS AND PRACTICES

"SEC. 1311. (a) In the case of any entity—

"(1) which cannot do business as a health maintenance organization in a State in which it proposes to furnish basic and supplemental health services because that State by law, regulation, or otherwise—

"(A) requires as a condition to doing business in that State that a medical society approve the furnishing of services by the entity,

"(B) requires that physicians constitute all or a percentage of its governing body,

"(C) requires that all physicians or a percentage of physicians in the locale participate or be permitted to participate in the provision of services for the entity, or

"(D) requires that the entity meet requirements for insurers of health care services doing business in that State respecting initial capitalization and establishment of financial reserves against insolvency, and

"(2) for which a grant, contract, loan, or loan guarantee was made under this title or which is a qualified health maintenance organization for purposes of section 1310 (relating to employees' health benefits plans),

such requirements shall not apply to that entity so as to prevent it from operating as a health maintenance organization in accordance with section 1301.

"(b) No State may establish or enforce any law which prevents a health maintenance organization for which a grant, contract, loan, or loan guarantee was made under this title or which is a qualified health maintenance organization for purposes of section 1310 (relating to employees' health benefits plans), from soliciting members through advertising its services, charges, or other nonprofessional aspects of its operation. This subsection does not authorize any advertising which identifies, refers to, or makes any qualitative judgment concerning, any health professional who provides services for a health maintenance organization.

"CONTINUED REGULATION OF HEALTH MAINTENANCE ORGANIZATIONS

"SEC. 1312. (a) If the Secretary determines that an entity which received a grant, contract, loan, or loan guarantee under this title as a health maintenance organization or which was included in a health benefits plan offered to employees pursuant to section 1310—

"(1) fails to provide basic and supplemental services to its members,

"(2) fails to provide such services in the manner prescribed by section 1301(b), or

"(3) is not organized or operated in the manner prescribed by section 1301(c),

the Secretary may, in addition to any other remedies available to him, bring a civil action in the United States district court for the district in which such entity is located to enforce its compliance with any assurances it furnished him respecting the provision of basic and supplemental health services or its organization or operation, as the case may be, which assurances were made under section 1310 or when application was made under this title for a grant, contract, loan, or loan guarantee.

"(b) The Secretary, through the Assistant Secretary for Health, shall administer subsection (a) in the Office of the Assistant Secretary for Health.

"LIMITATION ON SOURCE OF FUNDING FOR HEALTH MAINTENANCE ORGANIZATIONS

"SEC. 1313. No funds appropriated under any provision of this Act other than this title may be used—

"(1) for grants or contracts for surveys or other activities to determine the feasibility of developing or expanding health maintenance organizations or other entities which provide, directly or indirectly, health services to a defined population on a prepaid basis;

"(2) for grants or contracts, or for payments under loan guarantees, for planning projects for the establishment or expansion of such organizations or entities;

"(3) for grants or contracts, or for payments under loan guarantees, for projects for the initial development or expansion of such organizations or entities; or

"(4) for loans, or for payments under loan guarantees, to assist in meeting the costs of the initial operation after establishment or expansion of such organizations or entities.

"PROGRAM EVALUATION

"SEC. 1314. (a) The Comptroller General shall evaluate the operations of at least fifty of the health maintenance organizations for which assistance was provided under section 1303, 1304, or 1305. The period of operation of such health maintenance organizations which shall be evaluated under this subsection shall be not less than thirty-six months. The Comptroller General shall report to the Congress the results of the evaluation not later than ninety days after at least fifty of such health maintenance organizations have been in operation for at least thirty-six months. Such report shall contain findings— *Report to Congress.*

"(1) with respect to the ability of the organizations evaluated to operate on a fiscally sound basis without continued Federal financial assistance,

"(2) with respect to the ability of such organizations to meet the requirements of section 1301(c) respecting their organization and operation,

"(3) with respect to the ability of such organizations to provide basic and supplemental health services in the manner prescribed by section 1301(b),

"(4) with respect to the ability of such organizations to include indigent and high-risk individuals in their membership, and

"(5) with respect to the ability of such organizations to provide services to medically underserved populations.

87 STAT. 933

Study.

"(b) The Comptroller General shall also conduct a study of the economic effects on employers resulting from their compliance with the requirements of section 1310. The Comptroller General shall report to the Congress the results of such study not later than thirty-six months after the date of the enactment of this title.

"(c) The Comptroller General shall evaluate (1) the operations of distinct categories of health maintenance organizations in comparison with each other, (2) health maintenance organizations as a group in comparison with alternative forms of health care delivery, and (3) the impact that health maintenance organizations, individually, by category, and as a group, have on the health of the public. The Comptroller General shall report to the Congress the results of such evaluation not later than thirty-six months after the date of the enactment of this title.

Report to Congress.

"ANNUAL REPORT

Review, report to Congress.

"SEC. 1315. (a) The Secretary shall periodically review the programs of assistance authorized by this title and make an annual report to the Congress of a summary of the activities under each program. The Secretary shall include in such summary—

"(1) a summary of each grant, contract, loan, or loan guarantee made under this title in the period covered by the report and a list of the health maintenance organizations which during such period became qualified health maintenance organizations for purposes of section 1310;

"(2) the statistics and other information reported in such period to the Secretary in accordance with section 1301(c)(11);

"(3) findings with respect to the ability of the health maintenance organizations assisted under this title—

"(A) to operate on a fiscally sound basis without continued Federal financial assistance,

"(B) to meet the requirements of section 1301(c) respecting their organization and operation,

"(C) to provide basic and supplemental health services in the manner prescribed by section 1301(b),

"(D) to include indigent and high-risk individuals in their membership, and

"(E) to provide services to medically underserved populations; and

"(4) findings with respect to—

"(A) the operation of distinct categories of health maintenance organizations in comparison with each other,

"(B) health maintenance organizations as a group in comparison with alternative forms of health care delivery, and

"(C) the impact that health maintenance organizations, individually, by category, and as a group, have on the health of the public.

Review.

"(b) The Office of Management and Budget may review the Secretary's report under subsection (a) before its submission to the Congress, but the Office may not revise the report or delay its submission, and it may submit to the Congress its comments (and those of other departments or agencies of the Government) respecting such report."

Comments, submittal to Congress.

QUALITY ASSURANCE

58 Stat. 691;
85 Stat. 65.
42 USC 241.

SEC. 3. Title III of the Public Health Service Act is amended by adding at the end thereof the following new part:

- 21 -

"Part K—Quality Assurance

"QUALITY ASSURANCE

"Sec. 399c. (a)(1) The Secretary, through the Assistant Secretary for Health, shall conduct research and evaluation programs respecting the effectiveness, administration, and enforcement of quality assurance programs. Such research and evaluation programs shall be carried out in cooperation with the entity within the Department which administers the programs of assistance under section 304. *Research and evaluation programs.*

"(2) For the purpose of carrying out paragraph (1), there are authorized to be appropriated $4,000,000 for the fiscal year ending June 30, 1974, $8,000,000 for the fiscal year ending June 30, 1975, $9,000,000 for the fiscal year ending June 30, 1976, $9,000,000 for the fiscal year ending June 30, 1977, and $10,000,000 for the fiscal year ending June 30, 1978. *81 Stat. 534. 42 USC 242b. Appropriation.*

"(b) The Secretary shall make an annual report to the Congress and the President on (1) the quality of health care in the United States, (2) the operation of quality assurance programs, and (3) advances made through research and evaluation of the effectiveness, administration, and enforcement of quality assurance programs. The first annual report under this subsection shall be made with respect to calendar year 1974 and shall be submitted not later than March 1, 1975. The Office of Management and Budget may review the Secretary's report under this subsection before its submission to the Congress, but the Office may not revise the report or delay its submission to the Congress, and it may submit to the Secretary and the Congress its comments (and those of other departments and agencies of the Government) with respect to such report." *Annual report to President and Congress.*

HEALTH CARE QUALITY ASSURANCE PROGRAMS STUDY

Sec. 4. (a) The Secretary of Health, Education, and Welfare shall contract, in accordance with subsection (b), for the conduct of a study to—

(1) analyze past and present mechanisms (both required by law and voluntary) to assure the quality of health care, identify the strengths and weaknesses of current major prototypes of health care quality assurance systems, and identify on a comparable basis the costs of such prototypes;

(2) provide a set of basic principles to be followed by any effective health care quality assurance system, including principles affecting the scope of the system, methods for assessing care, data requirements, specifications for the development of criteria and standards which relate to desired outcomes of care, and means for assessing the responsiveness of such care to the needs and perceptions of the consumers of such care;

(3) provide an assessment of programs for improving the performance of health practitioners and institutions in providing high-quality health care, including a study of the effectiveness of sanctions and educational programs;

(4) define the specific needs for a program of research and evaluation in health care quality assurance methods, including the design of prospective evaluations protocols for health care quality assurance systems; and

(5) provide methods for assessing the quality of health care from the point of view of consumers of such care.

(b) The Secretary shall contract for the conduct of the study required by subsection (a) with a nonprofit private organization which— *Contract with private organization.*

(1) has a national reputation for objectivity in the conduct of studies for the Federal Government;

(2) has the capacity to readily marshall the widest possible range of expertise and advice relevant to the conduct of such study;

(3) has a membership and competent staff which have backgrounds in government, the health sciences, and the social sciences;

(4) has a history of interest and activity in health policy issues related to such study; and

(5) has extensive existing contracts with interested public and private agencies and organizations.

The Secretary shall enter into such contract within 90 days of the date of the enactment of the first Act making an appropriation under subsection (d).

Reports to congressional committees.

(c) An interim report providing a plan for the study required by subsection (a) shall be submitted by the organization conducting the study to the Committee on Interstate and Foreign Commerce of the House of Representatives and the Committee on Labor and Public Welfare of the Senate by June 30, 1974; and a final report giving the results of the study and providing specifications for an effective quality assurance system shall be submitted by such organization to the Committee on Interstate and Foreign Commerce of the House of Representatives and the Committee on Labor and Public Welfare of the Senate by January 31, 1976.

Appropriation.

(d) There is authorized to be appropriated $10,000,000, which shall be available without fiscal year limitation, for the conduct of the study required by subsection (a).

REPORTS RESPECTING MEDICALLY UNDERSERVED AREAS AND POPULATION GROUPS AND NON-METROPOLITAN AREAS

Reports to Congress.

Ante, p. 917.

Review.

Comments, submittal to Congress.

SEC. 5. Within three months of the date of the enactment of this Act, the Secretary of Health, Education, and Welfare shall report to the Congress the criteria used by him in the designation of medically underserved areas and population groups for the purposes of section 1302(7) of the Public Health Service Act. Within one year of such date, the Secretary shall report to the Congress (1) the areas and population groups designated by him under such section 1302(7) as having a shortage of personal health services, (2) the comments (if any) submitted by State and areawide comprehensive health planning agencies under such section with respect to any such designation, and (3) the areas which meet the definitional standards under section 1302(9) of such Act for non-metropolitan areas. The Office of Management and Budget may review the Secretary's report under this section before its submission to the Congress, but the Office may not revise the report or delay its submission beyond the date prescribed for its submission, and it may submit to Congress its comments (and those of other departments and agencies of the Government) respecting such report.

HEALTH SERVICES FOR INDIANS AND DOMESTIC AGRICULTURAL MIGRATORY AND SEASONAL WORKERS

68 Stat. 674.

SEC. 6. (a) The first section of the Act of August 5, 1954 (42 U.S.C. 2001), is amended by inserting "(a)" after "That" and by adding at the end thereof the following new subsection:

"(b) In carrying out his functions, responsibilities, authorities, and duties under this Act, the Secretary is authorized, with the consent of the Indian people served, to contract with private or other non-

87 STAT. 936

Federal health agencies or organizations for the provision of health services to such people on a fee-for-service basis or on a prepayment or other similar basis.".

(b) The Secretary of Health, Education, and Welfare, in connection with existing authority (except section 310 of the Public Health Service Act) for the provision of health services to domestic agricultural migratory workers, to persons who perform seasonal agricultural services similar to the services performed by such workers, and to the families of such workers and persons, is authorized to arrange for the provision of health services to such workers and persons and their families through health maintenance organizations. In carrying out this subsection the Secretary may only use sums appropriated after the date of the enactment of this Act.

76 Stat. 592.
42 USC 242h.

CONFORMING AMENDMENTS

SEC. 7. (a) Section 1 of the Public Health Service Act is amended to read as follows:

58 Stat. 682;
86 Stat. 137.
42 USC 201 note.

"SHORT TITLE

"SECTION 1. This Act may be cited as the 'Public Health Service Act'."

(b) Title XIII of the Act of July 1, 1944 (58 Stat. 682) (as so designated by section 2(b) of the Emergency Medical Services Systems Act of 1973 (Public Law 93–154)) is repealed.

Repeal.

Ante, p. 604.

(c) Section 306(g) of the Federal National Mortgage Association Act (12 U.S.C. 1721(g)) is amended by inserting ", or which are guaranteed under title XIII of the Pubic Health Service Act" after "chapter 37 of title 38, United States Code".

82 Stat. 542.

38 USC 1801.

Approved December 29, 1973.

LEGISLATIVE HISTORY:

HOUSE REPORTS: No. 93-451 accompanying H. R. 7974 (Comm. on
                Interstate and Foreign Commerce) and No. 93-714
                (Comm. of Conference).
SENATE REPORTS: No. 93-129 (Comm. on Labor and Public Welfare) and
                No. 93-621 (Comm. of Conference).
CONGRESSIONAL RECORD, Vol. 119 (1973):
    May 14, 15, considered and passed Senate.
    Sept. 12, considered and passed House, amended, in lieu of
        H. R. 7974.
    Dec. 18, House agreed to conference report.
    Dec. 19, Senate agreed to conference report.
WEEKLY COMPILATION OF PRESIDENTIAL DOCUMENTS, Vol. 10, No. 1 (1974):
    Dec. 29, 1973, Presidential statement.

○

Appendix B

HEALTH MAINTENANCE ORGANIZATION MODEL ACT

Reprinted with the permission of the National Association of Insurance Commissioners (NAIC)

Table of Contents

Section 1.   Short Title
Section 2.   Definitions
Section 3.   Establishment of Health Maintenance Organizations
Section 4.   Issuance of Certificate of Authority
Section 5.   Powers of Health Maintenance Organizations
Section 6.   Fiduciary Responsibilities
Section 7.   Quality Assurance Program
Section 8.   Requirements for Group Contract, Individual Contract and Evidence of Coverage
Section 9.   Annual Report
Section 10. Information to Enrollees or Subscribers
Section 11. Grievance Procedures
Section 12. Investments
Section 13. Protection Against Insolvency
Section 14. Uncovered Expenditures Insolvency Deposit
Section 15. Enrollment Period, Replacement Coverage in the Event of Insolvency
Section 16. Filing Requirements for Rating Information
Section 17. Regulation of Health Maintenance Organization Producers
Section 18. Powers of Insurers and [Hospital and Medical Service Corporations]
Section 19. Examinations
Section 20. Suspension or Revocation of Certificate of Authority
Section 21. Rehabilitation, Liquidation or Conservation of Health Maintenance Organizations
Section 22. Summary Orders and Supervision
Section 23. Regulations
Section 24. Fees
Section 25. Penalties and Enforcement
Section 26. Statutory Construction and Relationship to Other Laws
Section 27. Filings and Reports as Public Documents
Section 28. Confidentiality of Medical Information and Limitation of Liability
Section 29. [Commissioner of Public Health's] Authority to Contract
Section 30. Acquisition of Control of or Merger of a Health Maintenance Organization
Section 31. Dual Choice [optional]
Section 32. Coordination of Benefits
Section 33. Insolvency Protection; Assessment
Section 34. Severability

Section 1. Short Title

This Act may be cited as the Health Maintenance Organization Act of [insert year].

Introductory Comment:

Nature of the Health Maintenance Organization

A health maintenance organization may be described as an organization which brings together a comprehensive range of medical services in a single organization to assure a patient of convenient access to health care services. It furnishes needed services for a prepaid fixed fee paid by or on behalf of the enrollees. An HMO can be organized, operated and financed in a variety of ways. For example, an HMO may be organized by physicians, hospitals, community groups, labor unions, government units, insurance companies, etc. Generally speaking, an HMO delivery system is predicated on three principles: (1) It is an organized system for the delivery of health care which brings together health care providers; (2) Such an arrangement makes available basic health care which the enrolled group might reasonably require, including emphasis on the prevention of illness or disability; (3) The payments will be made on a prepayment basis, whether by the individual enrollees, Medicare, Medicaid or through employer-employee arrangements.

How might the HMO concept contribute to alleviating the difficulties posed by the current health care delivery system?

An HMO can directly address itself to the problems of availability, accessibility and continuity, since it is a health care delivery system. It assumes responsibility for actually furnishing to its enrollees those health care services necessary to meet the obligations it undertakes. Thus the HMO occupies a position through which both the accessibility and continuity of care may be affected.

An HMO, by its very nature, may provide incentives toward lessening costs in delivering health care. It has a limited membership prepaying fixed sums of money. The providers are obligated to deliver a specified set of health care services. The fixed amount of income provides incentive to control expenses and costs. The HMO provides a mechanism to analyze costs, expenses and utilization of services, and affords a means to implement measures to enhance efficiency.

The problem of the quality of health care is not susceptible to an easy solution. An HMO is in a position to assess the quality of care provided since it is a closed system. It can study the health of its members, review the records of treatment and, in general, provide a monitoring mechanism.

The Need for State Authorizing and Regulatory Legislation

From 1970 to 1973, the administration and committees in both houses of Congress spent much time analyzing the health maintenance organization alternative in connection with national health insurance and federal assistance bills for HMOs. This analysis resulted in the enactment of the federal HMO Act in 1973. Since then, the number of health maintenance organizations and the number of HMO enrollees has grown rapidly. Prior to 1972, however, few states had a statutory framework tailored to the supervision of health maintenance organizations. Chartering, licensing, contract and rate regulation, and other supervision was being carried out under general insurance laws, hospital and medical service corporation statutes, other special statutes, or not at all. Because the HMO is a unique type of organization, many provisions of such state laws were inapplicable highly restrictive or prohibitive to the formation and operation of an HMO. Therefore, in 1972 the NAIC adopted the Model Health Maintenance Organization Act which accommodates the unique features of HMOs.

Purpose of a State Model Bill

The model bill clearly authorizes the establishment and operation of HMOs. Restrictive provisions in other laws which are inappropriate to HMOs are rendered inapplicable. Appropriate grants of authority are established to enable the HMOs to fulfill the function envisioned for them. At the same time, however, the public has a vital interest in the fiscally sound, efficient and ethical operation of HMOs. As is the case with insurance and hospital and medical service corporations, HMOs are "affected with the public interest." Regulatory safeguards dovetailed to the unique nature of HMOs are essential. Thus, the purpose of this model bill is twofold.

First, it attempts to provide a legal framework enabling the organization and functioning of HMOs of a wide variety including those based upon the medical care foundation or individual practice association concept. The legal environment is designed to permit a high degree of flexibility. No one form of organization or one type of modus operandi is required. Instead the HMO concept can be refined and subjected to further experimentation. Second, the model bill attempts to provide a regulatory monitoring system not only to prevent or remedy abuse, but also to assist in the future improvement and development of this alternative form of a health care delivery system.

Of course, it is also possible that the statutes of a given state are presently broad enough to allow operation of at least certain types of HMOs and provide the commissioner with appropriate authority to regulate them. In those states, a bill such as this may be desirable in order to consolidate and define more clearly the authority for and manner of regulation of an HMO. However, it may be possible to form HMOs under existing laws in some states before passage of this model legislation and it is anticipated that such programs can develop concurrently with any legislative activity.

The model, or substantial portions of it, has been enacted in 27 states and substantial experience has been gained in implementing and regulating HMOs under its terms. In addition, as HMOs have become insolvent and commissioners have had to deal with the results of those insolvencies, the model act has been revised to reflect changes which have occurred in the federal law, to reflect experience gained in administering the law, and to clarify and strengthen the provisions relating to HMO solvency.

It may be necessary to modify or replace certain language in the model bill prior to legislative consideration to make terminology consistent with existing law in a particular state. To simplify this adjustment, three frequently used terms known to be subject to variation from state to state are enclosed in brackets wherever used in order to facilitate necessary modification. These terms are: (1) commissioner, whose counterparts in some states are known as director or superintendent; (2) commissioner of public health, whose counterparts in other states are known as director of public health or by some other title; and (3) hospital or medical service corporations, whose counterparts in other states may be known as health service corporations, hospital indemnity corporations, etc. Where specific reference to existing state laws is required, the nature of the citation is indicated in brackets.

The model bill provides that the principal regulator is the commissioner of insurance. It may be desirable for the commissioner to have an advisory council to advise him in carrying out his duties under the Act. Such an advisory council could be established through the promulgation of a regulation pursuant to Section 23 of the model bill or by adding a new section to the model bill.

Section 2. Definitions

A. "Basic health care services" means the following medically necessary services: preventive care, emergency care, inpatient and outpatient hospital and physician care, diagnostic laboratory and diagnostic and therapeutic radiological services. It does not include mental health services or services for alcohol or drug abuse, dental or vision services or long-term rehabilitation treatment.

B. "Capitated basis" means fixed per member per month payment or percentage of premium payment wherein the provider assumes the full risk for the cost of contracted services without regard to the type, value or frequency of services provided. For purposes of this definition, capitated basis includes the cost associated with operating staff model facilities.

C. "Carrier" shall mean a health maintenance organization, an insurer, a nonprofit hospital and medical service corporation, or other entity responsible for the payment of benefits or provision of services under a group contract.

D. "Commissioner" [director, superintendent] means the commissioner [director, superintendent] of insurance.

E. "Copayment" means an amount an enrollee must pay in order to receive a specific service which is not fully prepaid.

F. "Deductible" means the amount an enrollee is responsible to pay out-of-pocket before the health maintenance organization begins to pay the costs associated with treatment.

G. "Enrollee" means an individual who is covered by a health maintenance organization.

H. "Evidence of coverage" means a statement of the essential features and services of the health maintenance organization coverage which is given to the subscriber by the health maintenance organization or by the group contract holder.

I. "Extension of benefits" shall mean the continuation of coverage under a particular benefit provided under a contract following termination with respect to an enrollee who is totally disabled on the date of termination.

J. "Grievance" means a written complaint submitted in accordance with the health maintenance organization's formal grievance procedure by or on behalf of the enrollee regarding any aspect of the health maintenance organization relative to the enrollee.

K. "Group contract" means a contract for health care services which by its terms limits eligibility to members of a specified group. The group contract may include coverage for dependents.

L. "Group contract holder" means the person to which a group contract has been issued.

M. "Health maintenance organization" means any person that undertakes to provide or arrange for the delivery of basic health care services to enrollees on a prepaid basis, except for enrollee responsibility for copayments and/or deductibles.

N. "Health maintenance organization producer" means a person who solicits, negotiates, effects, procures, delivers, renews or continues a policy or contract for HMO membership, or who takes or transmits a membership fee or premium for such a policy or contract, other than for himself, or a person who advertises or otherwise holds himself out to the public as such.

O. "Individual contract" means a contract for health care services issued to and covering an individual. The individual contract may include dependents of the subscriber.

P. "Insolvent" or "Insolvency" shall mean that the organization has been declared insolvent and placed under an order of liquidation by a court of competent jurisdiction.

Q. "Managed hospital payment basis" means agreements wherein the financial risk is primarily related to the degree of utilization rather than to the cost of services.

Comment: Examples of Subsection Q agreements include but are not limited to payments on a DRG or per diem basis or where there is an agreement between a hospital and health maintenance organization which are under common ownership or control.

R. "Net worth" means the excess of total admitted assets over total liabilities, but the liabilities shall not include fully subordinated debt.

S. "Participating provider" means a provider as defined in U below who, under an express or implied contract with the health maintenance organization or with its contractor or subcontractor, has agreed to provide health care services to enrollees with an expectation of receiving payment, other than copayment or deductible, directly or indirectly from the health maintenance organization.

T. "Person" means any natural or artificial person including but not limited to individuals, partnerships, associations, trusts or corporations.

U. "Provider" means any physician, hospital or other person licensed or otherwise authorized to furnish health care services.

V. "Replacement coverage" shall mean the benefits provided by a succeeding carrier.

W. "Subscriber" means an individual whose employment or other status, except family depen-

dency, is the basis for eligibility for enrollment in the health maintenance organization, or
in the case of an individual contract, the person in whose name the contract is issued.

X. "Uncovered expenditures" means the costs to the health maintenance organization for
health care services that are the obligation of the health maintenance organization, for
which an enrollee may also be liable in the event of the health maintenance organization's insolvency and for which no alternative arrangements have been made that are
acceptable to the commissioner [director, superintendent].

Comment: Subsection X defines uncovered expenditures for use in Section 13. They will
vary in type and amount, depending on the arrangements of the HMO. They may include
out-of-area services, referral services and hospital services. They do not include expenditures
for services when a provider has agreed not to bill the enrollee even though the provider is
not paid by the HMO, or for services that are guaranteed, insured or assumed by a person or
organization other than the health maintenance organization.

Section 3. Establishment of Health Maintenance Organizations

A. Notwithstanding any law of this state to the contrary, any person may apply to the commissioner [director, superintendent] for a certificate of authority to establish and operate a
health maintenance organization in compliance with this Act. No person shall establish or
operate a health maintenance organization in this state, without obtaining a certificate of
authority under this Act. A foreign corporation may qualify under this Act, subject to its
registration to do business in this state as a foreign corporation under [insert citation] and
compliance with all provisions of this Act and other applicable state laws.

B. Any health maintenance organization which has not previously received a certificate of authority to operate as a health maintenance organization as of the effective date of this Act
shall submit an application for a certificate of authority under Subsection C within [insert
number] days of the effective date of this Act. Each such applicant may continue to operate until the commissioner [director, superintendent] acts upon the application. In the
event that an application is denied under Section 4, the applicant shall thereafter be
treated as a health maintenance organization whose certificate of authority has been revoked.

C. Each application for a certificate of authority shall be verified by an officer or authorized
representative of the applicant, shall be in a form prescribed by the commissioner [direc-
tor, superintendent], and shall set forth or be accompanied by the following:

  (1) A copy of the organizational documents of the applicant, such as the articles of in-
  corporation, articles of association, partnership agreement, trust agreement, or other
  applicable documents, and all amendments thereto;

  (2) A copy of the bylaws, rules and regulations, or similar document, if any, regulating
  the conduct of the internal affairs of the applicant;

  (3) A list of the names, addresses and official positions and biographical information on
  forms acceptable to the commissioner [director, superintendent] of the persons who
  are to be responsible for the conduct of the affairs and day to day operations of the

applicant, including all members of the board of directors, board of trustees, executive committee or other governing board or committee and the principal officers in the case of a corporation, or the partners or members in the case of a partnership or association;

Comment: NAIC biographical forms are recommended.

(4) A copy of any contract form made or to be made between any class of providers and the health maintenance organization and a copy of any contract made or to be made between third party administrators, marketing consultants or persons listed in Paragraph (3) and the health maintenance organization;

(5) A copy of the form of evidence of coverage to be issued to the enrollees;

(6) A copy of the form of group contract, if any, which is to be issued to employers, unions, trustees or other organizations;

(7) Financial statements showing the applicant's assets, liabilities and sources of financial support. Include both a copy of the applicant's most recent (regular) certified financial statement and an unaudited current financial statement;

(8) A financial feasibility plan which includes detailed enrollment projections, the methodology for determining premium rates to be charged during the first twelve months of operations certified by an actuary or other qualified person, a projection of balance sheets, cash flow statements showing any capital expenditures, purchase and sale of investments and deposits with the state, and income and expense statements anticipated from the start of operations until the organization has had net income for at least one year, and a statement as to the sources of working capital as well as any other sources of funding;

(9) A power of attorney duly executed by such applicant, if not domiciled in this state, appointing the commissioner [director, superintendent] and his successors in office, and duly authorized deputies, as the true and lawful attorney of such applicant in and for this state upon whom all lawful process in any legal action or proceeding against the health maintenance organization on a cause of action arising in this state may be served;

(10) A statement or map reasonably describing the geographic area or areas to be served;

(11) A description of the internal grievance procedures to be utilized for the investigation and resolution of enrollee complaints and grievances;

(12) A description of the proposed quality assurance program, including the formal organizational structure, methods for developing criteria, procedures for comprehensive evaluation of the quality of care rendered to enrollees, and processes to initiate corrective action and reevaluation when deficiencies in provider or organizational performance are identified;

(13) A description of the procedures to be implemented to meet the protection against insolvency requirements in Section 13;

(14) A list of the names, addresses, and license numbers of all providers with which the health maintenance organization has agreements;

(15) Such other information as the commissioner [director, superintendent] may require to make the determinations required in Section 4.

D. (1) The commissioner [director, superintendent] may promulgate such rules and regulations as he deems necessary to the proper administration of this Act to require a health maintenance organization, subsequent to receiving its certificate of authority, to submit the information, modifications or amendments to the items described in Subsection C of this section to the commissioner [director, superintendent], either for his approval or for information only, prior to the effectuation of the modification or amendment, or to require the health maintenance organization to indicate the modifications to both [the commissioner of public health] and the commissioner [director, superintendent] at the time of the next succeeding site visit or examination.

(2) Any modification or amendment for which the commissioner's [director's, superintendent's] approval is required shall be deemed approved unless disapproved within thirty (30) days, provided that the commissioner [director, superintendent] may postpone the action for such further time, not exceeding an additional thirty (30) days, as necessary for proper consideration.

Comment: Section 3 requires the licensing of an HMO in order to provide health care services on a prepaid basis. The legal entity, in which the responsibilities imposed by this Act are vested, serves as the focus of regulatory attention to assure that the consuming public is well served.

Subsection A is intended to provide a general override to existing state laws which restrict or prevent the formation or operation of health maintenance organizations. Among other restrictions, existing state laws may:

(1) Require approval of a health maintenance organization by a medical society;

(2) Require that physicians constitute all or a majority of the governing body of a health maintenance organization;

(3) Require that all physicians or a percentage of physicians in the local medical society be permitted to participate in rendering the services of the organization;

(4) Require that such organization submit to regulation as an insurer of health care services;

(5) Require that only unincorporated individuals or associations or partnerships may provide health care services;

(6) Prohibit advertising by a professional group for recruitment of enrollees.

In addition to the general override provided in Subsection A, Section 26 specifically provides that the insurance law, the hospital and medical service corporation law and certain other provisions do not apply to HMOs.

It is assumed that, restrictive provisions of state law having been overcome, the "person" making application for a certificate of authority, if not an individual, will be created through existing state mechanisms such as the applicable nonprofit corporation act, business corporation act, etc. as appropriate. Since state laws generally establish detailed procedures related to business organizations, inclusion of organizational procedures in a model act of this nature would appear unnecessary. A business having incorporated under the law of a foreign state could qualify under this act after following appropriate state procedures required of foreign corporations seeking to do business in the state.

Section 4. Issuance of Certificate of Authority

A. (1) Upon receipt of an application for issuance of a certificate of authority, the commissioner [director, superintendent] shall forthwith transmit copies of such application and accompanying documents to the [commissioner of public health].

(2) The [commissioner of public health] shall determine whether the applicant for a certificate of authority, with respect to health care services to be furnished has complied with Section 7 of this Act.

(3) Within forty-five (45) days of receipt of the application for issuance of a certificate of authority, the [commissioner of public health] shall certify to the commissioner [director, superintendent] that the proposed health maintenance organization meets the requirements of Section 7 or notify the commissioner [director, superintendent] that the health maintenance organization does not meet such requirements and specify in what respects it is deficient.

B. The commissioner [director, superintendent] shall within forty-five (45) days of receipt of certification or notice of deficiencies from the [commissioner of public health] issue a certificate of authority to any person filing a completed application upon receiving the prescribed fees and upon the commissioner [director, superintendent] being satisfied that:

(1) The persons responsible for the conduct of the affairs of the applicant are competent, trustworthy and possess good reputations;

(2) Any deficiencies identified by the [commissioner of public health] have been corrected and the [commissioner of public health] has certified to the commissioner [director, superintendent] that the health maintenance organization's proposed plan of operation meets the requirements of Section 7;

(3) The health maintenance organization will effectively provide or arrange for the provision of basic health care services on a prepaid basis, through insurance or otherwise, except to the extent of reasonable requirements for copayments and/or deductibles; and

(4) The health maintenance organization is in compliance with Sections 13 and 15 of this Act.

C. A certificate of authority shall be denied only after the commissioner [director, superintendent] complies with the requirements of Section 20.

Comment: A health maintenance organization combines several characteristics of an insurance operation (including the need for financial responsibility, the assumption of risk and similarity in marketing activities) with the characteristics of a health care delivery system. Section 4 provides for the authorization and regulation of health maintenance organizations to be carried out through existing state agencies. The creation of a new agency specifically for health maintenance organizations would unnecessarily duplicate existing functions in the state insurance and health departments. It is felt that the expertise of the state insurance department on fiscal and other regulatory matters and the familiarity of the state health department with regard to health matters should both be utilized in the regulation of health maintenance organizations. To minimize administrative problems, the prime responsibility for administration is vested in one agency—the insurance department. However, to the extent possible, the responsibilities of the two agencies are clearly defined with the insurance commissioner obligated to rely on the health department with respect to the latter's sphere of expertise.

Comment: Subsection B(3) makes explicit the requirement that an health maintenance organization must provide a minimum package of services on a prepaid basis. Reasonable copayments, however, are permitted and do not violate the requirement for prepayment. Such copayments may be used to (1) reduce the amount of prepayments and (2) minimize frivolous utilization of services. In addition, an health maintenance organization may have more than one benefit package involving different levels of copayments.

Section 5. Powers of Health Maintenance Organizations

A. The powers of a health maintenance organization include, but are not limited to, the following:

(1) The purchase, lease, construction, renovation, operation or maintenance of hospitals, medical facilities, or both, and their ancillary equipment, and such property as may reasonably be required for its principal office or for such purposes as may be necessary in the transaction of the business of the organization;

(2) Transactions between affiliated entities, including loans and the transfer of responsibility under all contracts (provider, subscriber, etc.) between affiliates or between the health maintenance organization and its parent;

(3) The furnishing of health care services through providers, provider associations or agents for providers which are under contract with or employed by the health maintenance organization;

(4) The contracting with any person for the performance on its behalf of certain functions such as marketing, enrollment and administration;

(5) The contracting with an insurance company licensed in this state, or with a hospital or medical service corporation authorized to do business in this state, for the provision of insurance, indemnity or reimbursement against the cost of health care services provided by the health maintenance organization;

(6) The offering of other health care services, in addition to basic health care services. Non-basic health care services may be offered by a health maintenance organization

on a prepaid basis without offering basic health care services to any group or individual;

(7) The joint marketing of products with an insurance company licensed in this state or with a hospital or medical service corporation authorized to do business in this state as long as the company that is offering each product is clearly identified.

B. (1) A health maintenance organization shall file notice, with adequate supporting information, with the commissioner [director, superintendent] prior to the exercise of any power granted in Subsections A(1), (2) or (4) which may affect the financial soundness of the health maintenance organization. The commissioner [director, superintendent] shall disapprove such exercise of power only if in his opinion it would substantially and adversely affect the financial soundness of the health maintenance organization and endanger its ability to meet its obligations. If the commissioner [director, superintendent] does not disapprove within thirty (30) days of the filing, it shall be deemed approved.

(2) The commissioner [director, superintendent] may promulgate rules and regulations exempting from the filing requirement of Paragraph (1) those activities having a de minimis effect.

Section 6. Fiduciary Responsibilities

A. Any director, officer, employee or partner of a health maintenance organization who receives, collects, disburses or invests funds in connection with the activities of such organization shall be responsible for such funds in a fiduciary relationship to the organization.

B. A health maintenance organization shall maintain in force a fidelity bond or fidelity insurance on such employees and officers, directors and partners in an amount not less than $250,000 for each health maintenance organization or a maximum of $5,000,000 in aggregate maintained on behalf of health maintenance organizations owned by a common parent corporation, or such sum as may be prescribed by the commissioner [director, superintendent].

Comment: As an optional additional subsection, language may be included that would make the appropriate provisions of the state's insurance laws governing prohibitions or restrictions on activities of directors, officers and certain shareholders applicable to health maintenance organizations.

Section 7. Quality Assurance Program

A. The health maintenance organization shall establish procedures to assure that the health care services provided to enrollees shall be rendered under reasonable standards of quality of care consistent with prevailing professionally recognized standards of medical practice. Such procedures shall include mechanisms to assure availability, accessibility and continuity of care.

B. The health maintenance organization shall have an ongoing internal quality assurance program to monitor and evaluate its health care services, including primary and specialist physician services, and ancillary and preventive health care services, across all institutional and non-institutional settings. The program shall include, at a minimum, the following:

(1) A written statement of goals and objectives which emphasizes improved health status in evaluating the quality of care rendered to enrollees;

(2) A written quality assurance plan which describes the following:

(a) The health maintenance organization's scope and purpose in quality assurance;

(b) The organizational structure responsible for quality assurance activities;

(c) Contractual arrangements, where appropriate, for delegation of quality assurance activities;

(d) Confidentiality policies and procedures;

(e) A system of ongoing evaluation activities;

(f) A system of focused evaluation activities;

(g) A system for credentialing providers and performing peer review activities; and

(h) Duties and responsibilities of the designated physician responsible for the quality assurance activities;

(3) A written statement describing the system of ongoing quality assurance activities including:

(a) Problem assessment, identification, selection and study;

(b) Corrective action, monitoring, evaluation and reassessment; and

(c) Interpretation and analysis of patterns of care rendered to individual patients by individual providers;

(4) A written statement describing the system of focused quality assurance activities based on representative samples of the enrolled population which identifies method of topic selection, study, data collection, analysis, interpretation and report format; and

(5) Written plans for taking appropriate corrective action whenever, as determined by the quality assurance program, inappropriate or substandard services have been provided or services which should have been furnished have not been provided.

C. The organization shall record proceedings of formal quality assurance program activities and maintain documentation in a confidential manner. Quality assurance program minutes shall be available to the [commissioner of public health].

D. The organization shall ensure the use and maintenance of an adequate patient record system which will facilitate documentation and retrieval of clinical information for the purpose of the health maintenance organization evaluating continuity and coordination of patient care and assessing the quality of health and medical care provided to enrollees.

E. Enrollee clinical records shall be available to the [commissioner of public health] or an authorized designee for examination and review to ascertain compliance with this section, or as deemed necessary by the [commissioner of public health].

F. The organization shall establish a mechanism for periodic reporting of quality assurance program activities to the governing body, providers and appropriate organization staff.

Section 8. Requirements for Group Contract, Individual Contract and Evidence of Coverage

A. (1 Every group and individual contract holder is entitled to a group or individual contract.

(2 The contract shall not contain provisions or statements which are unjust, unfair, inequitable, misleading, deceptive, or which encourage misrepresentation as defined by [cite section of state law which implements the NAIC Unfair Trade Practices Act];

(3 The contract shall contain a clear statement of the following:

(a) Name and address of the health maintenance organization;

(b) Eligibility requirements;

(c) Benefits and services within the service area;

(d) Emergency care benefits and services;

(e) Out-of-area benefits and services (if any);

(f) Copayments, deductibles or other out-of-pocket expenses;

(g) Limitations and exclusions;

(h) Enrollee termination;

(i) Enrollee reinstatement (if any);

(j) Claims procedures;

(k) Enrollee grievance procedures;

(l) Continuation of coverage;

(m) Conversion;

(n) Extension of benefits (if any);

(o) Coordination of benefits (if applicable);

(p) Subrogation (if any);

(q) Description of the service area;

(r) Entire contract provision;

(s) Term of coverage;

(t) Cancellation of group or individual contract holder;

(u) Renewal;

(v) Reinstatement of group or individual contract holder (if any);

(w) Grace period; and

(x) Conformity with state law.

An evidence of coverage may be filed as part of the group contract to describe the provisions required in Paragraphs (3)(a) to (x) of this subsection.

B. In addition to those provisions required in Subsection A(3)(a) to (x), an individual contract shall provide for a ten-day period to examine and return the contract and have the premium refunded. If services were received during the ten-day period, and the person returns the contract to receive a refund of the premium paid, he or she must pay for such services.

C. (1) Every subscriber shall receive an evidence of coverage from the group contract holder or the health maintenance organization.

(2) The evidence of coverage shall not contain provisions or statements which are unfair, unjust, inequitable, misleading, deceptive, or which encourage misrepresentation as defined by [cite section of state law which implements the NAIC Unfair Trade Practices Act];

(3) The evidence of coverage shall contain a clear statement of the provisions required in Subsection A(3)(a) to (x).

D. The commissioner [director, superintendent] may adopt regulations establishing readability standards for individual contract, group contract, and evidence of coverage forms.

Comment: The commissioner [director, superintendent] may adopt standards provided for in the NAIC "Life and Health Insurance Policy Language Simplification Act."

E. No group or individual contract, evidence of coverage or amendment thereto, shall be delivered or issued for delivery in this state, unless its form has been filed with and approved by the commissioner [director, superintendent], subject to Subsections F and G of this section.

F. If an evidence of coverage issued pursuant to and incorporated in a contract issued in this state is intended for delivery in another state and the evidence of coverage has been approved for use in the state in which it is to be delivered, the evidence of coverage need not be submitted to the commissioner [director, superintendent] of this state for approval.

G. Every form required by Section 8 shall be filed with the commissioner [director, superintendent] not less than thirty (30) days prior to delivery or issue for delivery in this state. At any time during the initial thirty (30) day period, the commissioner [director, superintendent] may extend the period for review for an additional thirty (30) days. Notice of an extension shall be in writing. At the end of the review period, the form is deemed approved if the commissioner [director, superintendent] has taken no action. The filer must notify the commissioner [director, superintendent] in writing prior to using a form that is deemed approved.

At any time, after thirty (30) days notice and for cause shown, the commissioner [director, superintendent] may withdraw approval of any form, effective at the end of the thirty (30) days.

When a filing is disapproved or approval of a form is withdrawn, the commissioner [director, superintendent] shall give the health maintenance organization written notice of the reasons for disapproval and in the notice shall inform the health maintenance organization that within thirty (30) days of receipt of the notice the health maintenance organization may request a hearing. A hearing will be conducted within thirty (30) days after the commissioner [director, superintendent] has received the request for hearing.

H. The commissioner [director, superintendent] may require the submission of whatever relevant information he deems necessary in determining whether to approve or disapprove a filing made pursuant to this section.

Section 9. Annual Report

A. Every health maintenance organization shall annually, on or before the first day of March, file a report verified by at least two principal officers with the commissioner [director, superintendent], with a copy to the [commissioner of public health] covering the preceding calendar year. Such report shall be on forms prescribed by the commissioner [director, superintendent]. In addition, the health maintenance organization shall file by the first day of March, unless otherwise stated:

(1) Audited financial statements on or before June 1;

(2) A list of the providers who have executed a contract that complies with Section 13(D)(1) of this Act; and

(3) (a) A description of the grievance procedures, and

    (b) The total number of grievances handled through such procedures, a compilation of the causes underlying those grievances, and a summary of the final disposition of those grievances.

B. The commissioner [director, superintendent] may require such additional reports as are deemed necessary and appropriate to enable the commissioner [director, superintendent] to carry out his duties under this Act.

Section 10. Information to Enrollees or Subscribers

A. The health maintenance organization shall provide to its subscribers a list of providers, upon enrollment and re-enrollment.

B. Every health maintenance organization shall provide within thirty (30) days to its subscribers notice of any material change in the operation of the organization that will affect them directly.

C. An enrollee must be notified in writing by the health maintenance organization of the termination of the primary care provider who provided health care services to that enrollee. The health maintenance organization shall provide assistance to the enrollee in transferring to another participating primary care provider.

D. The health maintenance organization shall provide to subscribers information on how services may be obtained, where additional information on access to services can be obtained and a number where the enrollee can contact the HMO, at no cost to the enrollee.

Comment: For the purpose of this section any major change in the provider network is considered a material change.

Section 11. Grievance Procedures

A. Every health maintenance organization shall establish and maintain a grievance procedure which has been approved by the commissioner [director, superintendent], after consultation with the [commissioner of public health], to provide procedures for the resolution of grievances initiated by enrollees. The health maintenance organization shall maintain records regarding grievances received since the date of its last examination of such grievances.

B. The commissioner [director, superintendent] or the [commissioner of public health] may examine such grievance procedures.

Section 12. Investments

With the exception of investments made in accordance with Section 5A(1), the funds of a health maintenance organization shall be invested only in accordance with [cite section of law or regulation implementing the NAIC "Health Maintenance Organization Investment Guidelines."]

Section 13. Protection Against Insolvency

A. Net Worth Requirements

(1) Before issuing any certificate of authority, the commissioner [director, superintendent] shall require that the health maintenance organization have an initial net worth of one million five hundred thousand dollars ($1,500,000) and shall thereafter maintain the minimum net worth required under Paragraph (2).

(2) Except as provided in Paragraphs (3) and (4) of this subsection, every health maintenance organization must maintain a minimum net worth equal to the greater of:

(a) One million dollars ($1,000,000); or

(b) Two percent (2%) of annual premium revenues as reported on the most recent annual financial statement filed with the commissioner [director, superintendent] on the first $150,000,000 of premium and one percent of annual premium on the premium in excess of $150,000,000; or

(c) An amount equal to the sum of three months' uncovered health care expenditures as reported on the most recent financial statement filed with the commissioner [director, superintendent]; or

(d) An amount equal to the sum of:

    (i) Eight percent (8%) of annual health care expenditures except those paid on a capitated basis or managed hospital payment basis as reported on the most recent financial statement filed with the commissioner [director, superintendent]; and

    (ii) Four percent (4%) of annual hospital expenditures paid on a managed hospital payment basis as reported on the most recent financial statement filed with the commissioner [director, superintendent].

(3) A health maintenance organization licensed before the effective date of this Act must maintain a minimum net worth of:

(a) Twenty-five percent (25%) of the amount required by Section 13(A)(2) by December 31, 19__;

(b) Fifty percent (50%) of the amount required by Section 13(A)(2) by December 31, 19__;

(c) Seventy-five percent (75%) of the amount required by Section 13(A)(2) by December 31, 19__;

(d) One hundred percent (100%) of the amount required by Section 13(A)(2) by December 31, 19__.

(4) (a) In determining net worth, no debt shall be considered fully subordinated unless the subordination clause is in a form acceptable to the commissioner [director, superintendent]. Any interest obligation relating to the repayment of any subordinated debt must be similarly subordinated.

(b) The interest expenses relating to the repayment of any fully subordinated debt shall be considered covered expenses.

(c) Any debt incurred by a note meeting the requirements of this section, and otherwise acceptable to the commissioner [director, superintendent], shall not be considered a liability and shall be recorded as equity.

B. Deposit Requirements

(1) Unless otherwise provided below, each health maintenance organization shall deposit with the commissioner [director, superintendent] or, at the discretion of the commissioner [director, superintendent], with any organization or trustee acceptable to him through which a custodial or controlled account is utilized, cash, securities, or any

combination of these or other measures that are acceptable to him which at all times shall have a value of not less than three hundred thousand dollars ($300,000).

(2) A health maintenance organization that is in operation on the effective date of th_s section shall make a deposit equal to one hundred fifty thousand dollars ($150,0C0).

In the second year, the amount of the additional deposit for a health maintenance organization that is in operation on the effective date of the section shall be equal to one hundred fifty thousand dollars ($150,000), for a total of three hundred thousend dollars ($300,000).

(3) The deposit shall be an admitted asset of the health maintenance organization in the determination of net worth.

(4) All income from deposits shall be an asset of the organization. A health maintenance organization that has made a securities deposit may withdraw that deposit or any part thereof after making a substitute deposit of cash, securities, or any combination cf these or other measures of equal amount and value. Any securities shall be apprcved by the commissioner [director, superintendent] before being deposited or substitu:ed.

(5) The deposit shall be used to protect the interests of the health maintenance organization's enrollees and to assure continuation of health care services to enrollees of a health maintenance organization which is in rehabilitation or conservation. The commissioner [director, superintendent] may use the deposit for administrative costs directly attributable to a receivership or liquidation. If the health maintenance organization is placed in receivership or liquidation, the deposit shall be an asset subject to the provisions of the liquidation act.

(6) The commissioner [director, superintendent] may reduce or eliminate the deposit requirement if the health maintenance organization deposits with the state treasurer. insurance commissioner [director, superintendent], or other official body of the stat2 or jurisdiction of domicile for the protection of all subscribers and enrollees, whereer located, of such health maintenance organization, cash, acceptable securities or surety, and delivers to the commissioner [director, superintendent] a certificate to such effect, duly authenticated by the appropriate state official holding the deposit.

C. Liabilities

Every health maintenance organization shall, when determining liabilities, include an amount estimated in the aggregate to provide for any unearned premium and for the payment of all claims for health care expenditures which have been incurred, whether reported or unreported, which are unpaid and for which such organization is or may be liable, and to provide for the expense of adjustment or settlement of such claims.

Such liabilities shall be computed in accordance with regulations promulgated by the commissioner [director, superintendent] upon reasonable consideration of the ascertained experience and character of the health maintenance organization.

D. Hold Harmless

(1) Every contract between a health maintenance organization and a participating pro-

vider of health care services shall be in writing and shall set forth that in the event the health maintenance organization fails to pay for health care services as set forth in the contract, the subscriber or enrollee shall not be liable to the provider for any sums owed by the health maintenance organization.

(2) In the event that the participating provider contract has not been reduced to writing as required by this subsection or that the contract fails to contain the required prohibition, the participating provider shall not collect or attempt to collect from the subscriber or enrollee sums owed by the health maintenance organization.

(3) No participating provider, or agent, trustee or assignee thereof, may maintain any action at law against a subscriber or enrollee to collect sums owed by the health maintenance organization.

E. Continuation of Benefits

The commissioner [director, superintendent] shall require that each health maintenance organization have a plan for handling insolvency which allows for continuation of benefits for the duration of the contract period for which premiums have been paid and continuation of benefits to members who are confined on the date of insolvency in an inpatient facility until their discharge or expiration of benefits. In considering such a plan, the commissioner [director, superintendent] may require:

(1) Insurance to cover the expenses to be paid for continued benefits after an insolvency;

(2) Provisions in provider contracts that obligate the provider to provide services for the duration of the period after the health maintenance organization's insolvency for which premium payment has been made and until the enrollees' discharge from inpatient facilities;

(3) Insolvency reserves;

(4) Acceptable letters of credit;

(5) Any other arrangements to assure that benefits are continued as specified above.

F. Notice of Termination

An agreement to provide health care services between a provider and a health maintenance organization must require that if the provider terminates the agreement, the provider shall give the organization at least sixty (60) days' advance notice of termination.

Section 14. Uncovered Expenditures Insolvency Deposit

A. If at any time uncovered expenditures exceed ten percent (10%) of total health care expenditures, a health maintenance organization shall place an uncovered expenditures insolvency deposit with the commissioner [director, superintendent], or with any organization or trustee acceptable to the commissioner [director, superintendent] through which a custodial or controlled account is maintained, cash or securities that are acceptable to the commissioner. Such deposit shall at all times have a fair market value in an amount of 120% of the HMO's outstanding liability for uncovered expenditures for enrollees in this state, including incurred but not reported claims, and shall be calculated as of the first day of the month and maintained for the remainder of the month. If a health maintenance organization is not otherwise required to file a quarterly report, it shall file a report within forty-five (45) days of the end of the calendar quarter with information sufficient to demonstrate compliance with this section.

B. The deposit required under this section is in addition to the deposit required under Section 13 and is an admitted asset of the health maintenance organization in the determination of net worth. All income from such deposits or trust accounts shall be assets of the health maintenance organization and may be withdrawn from such deposit or account quarterly with the approval of the commissioner [director, superintendent].

C. A health maintenance organization that has made a deposit may withdraw that deposit or any part of the deposit if (1) a substitute deposit of cash or securities of equal amount and value is made, (2) the fair market value exceeds the amount of the required deposit, or (3) the required deposit under Subsection A is reduced or eliminated. Deposits, substitutions or withdrawals may be made only with the prior written approval of the commissioner [director, superintendent].

D. The deposit required under this section is in trust and may be used only as provided under this section. The commissioner [director, superintendent] may use the deposit of an insolvent health maintenance organization for administrative costs associated with administering the deposit and payment of claims of enrollees of this state for uncovered expenditures in this state. Claims for uncovered expenditures shall be paid on a pro rata basis based on assets available to pay such ultimate liability for incurred expenditures. Partial distribution may be made pending final distribution. Any amount of the deposit remaining shall be paid into the liquidation or receivership of the health maintenance organization.

E. The commissioner [director, superintendent] may by regulation prescribe the time, manner and form for filing claims under Subsection D.

F. The commissioner [director, superintendent] may by regulation or order require health maintenance organizations to file annual, quarterly or more frequent reports as he deems necessary to demonstrate compliance with this section. The commissioner [director, superintendent] may require that the reports include liability for uncovered expenditures as well as an audit opinion.

Section 15. Enrollment Period, Replacement Coverage in the Event of Insolvency

A. Enrollment Period

(1) In the event of an insolvency of a health maintenance organization, upon order of the commissioner [director, superintendent] all other carriers that participated in the enrollment process with the insolvent health maintenance organization at a group's last regular enrollment period shall offer such group's enrollees of the insolvent health maintenance organization a thirty-day enrollment period commencing upon the date of

insolvency. Each carrier shall offer such enrollees of the insolvent health maintenance organization the same coverages and rates that it had offered to the enrollees of the group at its last regular enrollment period.

(2) If no other carrier had been offered to some groups enrolled in the insolvent health maintenance organization, or if the commissioner [director, superintendent] determines that the other health benefit plan(s) lack sufficient health care delivery resources to assure that health care services will be available and accessible to all of the group enrollees of the insolvent health maintenance organization, then the commissioner [director, superintendent] shall allocate equitably the insolvent health maintenance organization's group contracts for such groups among all health maintenance organizations which operate within a portion of the insolvent health maintenance organization's service area, taking into consideration the health care delivery resources of each health maintenance organization. Each health maintenance organization to which a group or groups are so allocated shall offer such group or groups the health maintenance organization's existing coverage which is most similar to each group's coverage with the insolvent health maintenance organization at rates determined in accordance with the successor health maintenance organization's existing rating methodology.

(3) The commissioner [director, superintendent] shall also allocate equitably the insolvent health maintenance organization's nongroup enrollees which are unable to obtain other coverage among all health maintenance organizations which operate within a portion of the insolvent health maintenance organization's service area, taking into consideration the health care delivery resources of each such health maintenance organization. Each health maintenance organization to which nongroup enrollees are allocated shall offer such nongroup enrollees the health maintenance organization's existing coverage for individual or conversion coverage as determined by his type of coverage in the insolvent health maintenance organization at rates determined in accordance with the successor health maintenance organization's existing rating methodology. Successor health maintenance organizations which do not offer direct nongroup enrollment may aggregate all of the allocated nongroup enrollees into one group for rating and coverage purposes.

Comment: Amendments to the insurance code regulating indemnity carriers may be necessary to bring the insurance carriers into the jurisdiction of this provision.

B. Replacement Coverage

(1) "Discontinuance" shall mean the termination of the contract between the group contract holder and a health maintenance organization due to the insolvency of the health maintenance organization, and does not refer to the termination of any agreement between any individual enrollee and the health maintenance organization.

(2) Any carrier providing replacement coverage with respect to group hospital, medical or surgical expense or service benefits within a period of sixty (60) days from the date of discontinuance of a prior health maintenance organization contract or policy providing such hospital, medical or surgical expense or service benefits shall immediately cover all enrollees who were validly covered under the previous health maintenance

organization contract or policy at the date of discontinuance and who would otherwise be eligible for coverage under the succeeding carrier's contract, regardless of any provisions of the contract relating to active employment or hospital confinement or pregnancy.

(3) Except to the extent benefits for the condition would have been reduced or excluded under the prior carrier's contract or policy, no provision in a succeeding carrier's contract of replacement coverage which would operate to reduce or exclude benefits on the basis that the condition giving rise to benefits preexisted the effective date of the succeeding carrier's contract shall be applied with respect to those enrollees validly covered under the prior carrier's contract or policy on the date of discontinuance

Section 16. Filing Requirements for Rating Information

A. No premium rate may be used until either a schedule of premium rates or methodology for determining premium rates has been filed with and approved by the commissioner [director, superintendent].

B. Either a specific schedule of premium rates, or a methodology for determining premium rates, shall be established in accordance with actuarial principles for various categories of enrollees, provided that the premium applicable to an enrollee shall not be individually determined based on the status of his/her health. However, the premium rates shall not be excessive, inadequate or unfairly discriminatory. A certification by a qualified actuary or other qualified person acceptable to the commissioner [director, superintendent] as to the appropriateness of the use of the methodology, based on reasonable assumptions, shall accompany the filing along with adequate supporting information.

C. The commissioner [director, superintendent] shall approve the schedule of premium rates or methodology for determining premium rates if the requirements of Subsection B are met. If the commissioner [director, superintendent] disapproves such filing, he shall notify the health maintenance organization. In the notice, the commissioner [director, superintendent] shall specify the reasons for his disapproval. A hearing will be conducted within thirty (30) days after a request in writing by the person filing. If the commissioner [director, superintendent] does not take action on such schedule or methodology within thirty (30) days of the filing of such schedule or methodology, it shall be deemed approved.

Section 17. Regulation of Health Maintenance Organization Producers

A. The commissioner [director, superintendent] may, after notice and hearing, promulgate such rules and regulations as are necessary to provide for the licensing of health maintenance organization producers. Such rules shall establish:

(1) The requirements for licensure of resident health maintenance organization producers;

(2) The conditions for entering into reciprocal agreements with other jurisdictions for the licensure of nonresident health maintenance organization producers;

(3) Any examination, prelicensing or continuing education requirements;

(4) The requirements for registering and terminating the appointment of health maintenance organization producers;

(5) Any requirements for registering any assumed names or office locations in which an health maintenance organization producer does business;

(6) The conditions for health maintenance organization producer license renewal;

(7) The grounds for denial, refusal, suspension or revocation of an health maintenance organization producer's license;

(8) Any required fees for the licensing activities of health maintenance organization producers; and

(9) Any other requirement or procedure and any form as may be reasonably necessary to provide for the effective administration of the licensing of health maintenance organization producers under this section.

B. None of the following shall be required to hold a health maintenance organization producer license:

(1) Any regular salaried officer or employee of a health maintenance organization who devotes substantially all of his time to activities other than the taking or transmitting of applications or membership fees or premiums for health maintenance organization membership, or who receives no commission or other compensation directly dependent upon the business obtained and who does not solicit or accept from the public applications for health maintenance organization membership;

(2) Employers or their officers or employees or the trustees of any employee benefit plan to the extent that such employers, officers, employees or trustees are engaged in the administration or operation of any program of employee benefits involving the use of health maintenance organization memberships; provided that such employers, officers, employees or trustees are not in any manner compensated directly or indirectly by the health maintenance organization issuing such health maintenance organization memberships;

(3) Banks or their officers and employees to the extent that such banks, officers and employees collect and remit charges by charging same against accounts of depositors on the orders of such depositors; or

(4) Any person or the employee of any person who has contracted to provide administrative, management or health care services to a health maintenance organization and who is compensated for those services by the payment of an amount calculated as a percentage of the revenues, net income or profit of the health maintenance organization, if that method of compensation is the sole basis for subjecting that person or the employee of the person to this Act.

C. The commissioner [director, superintendent] may by rule exempt certain classes of persons from the requirement of obtaining a license:

(1) If the functions they perform do not require special competence, trustworthiness or the regulatory surveillance made possible by licensing; or

(2) If other existing safeguards make regulation unnecessary.

Section 18. Powers of Insurers and [Hospital and Medical Service Corporations]

A. An insurance company licensed in this state, or a hospital or medical service corporation authorized to do business in this state, may either directly or through a subsidiary or affiliate organize and operate a health maintenance organization under the provisions of this Act. Notwithstanding any other law which may be inconsistent herewith, any two or more such insurance companies, hospital or medical service corporations, or subsidiaries or affiliates thereof, may jointly organize and operate a health maintenance organization. The business of insurance is deemed to include the providing of health care by a health maintenance organization owned or operated by an insurer or a subsidiary thereof.

B. Notwithstanding any provision of insurance and hospital or medical service corporation laws [citations], an insurer or a hospital or medical service corporation may contract with a health maintenance organization to provide insurance or similar protection against the cost of care provided through health maintenance organizations and to provide coverage in the event of the failure of the health maintenance organization to meet its obligations.

The enrollees of a health maintenance organization constitute a permissible group under such laws. Among other things, under such contracts, the insurer or hospital or medical service corporation may make benefit payments to health maintenance organizations for health care services rendered by providers.

Section 19. Examinations

A. The commissioner [director, superintendent] may make an examination of the affairs of any health maintenance organization and providers with whom such organization has contracts, agreements or other arrangements as often as is reasonably necessary for the protection of the interests of the people of this state but not less frequently than once every three (3) years.

B. The [commissioner of public health] may make an examination concerning the quality assurance program of the health maintenance organization and of any providers with whom such organization has contracts, agreements or other arrangements as often as is reasonably necessary for the protection of the interests of the people of this state but not less frequently than once every three (3) years.

C. Every health maintenance organization and provider shall submit its books and records for such examinations and in every way facilitate the completion of the examination. For the purpose of examinations, the commissioner [director, superintendent] and the [commissioner of public health] may administer oaths to, and examine the officers and agents of, the health maintenance organization and the principals of such providers concerning their business.

D. The expenses of examinations under this section shall be assessed against the health maintenance organization being examined and remitted to the commissioner [director, superintendent] or the [commissioner of public health] for whom the examination is being conducted.

E. In lieu of such examination, the commissioner [director, superintendent] or [commissioner of public health] may accept the report of an examination made by the commissioner [director, superintendent] or [commissioner of public health] of another state.

Section 20. Suspension or Revocation of Certificate of Authority

A. Any certificate of authority issued under this Act may be suspended or revoked, and any application for a certificate of authority may be denied, if the commissioner [director, superintendent] finds that any of the conditions listed below exist:

    (1) The health maintenance organization is operating significantly in contravention of its basic organizational document or in a manner contrary to that described in any other information submitted under Section 3, unless amendments to such submissions have been filed with and approved by the commissioner [director, superintendent];

    (2) The health maintenance organization issues an evidence of coverage or uses a schedule of charges for health care services which do not comply with the requirements of Section 8 and 16;

    (3) The health maintenance organization does not provide or arrange for basic health care services;

    (4) The [commissioner of public health] certifies to the commissioner [director, superintendent] that:

        (a) The health maintenance organization does not meet the requirements of Section 4A(2); or

        (b) The health maintenance organization is unable to fulfill its obligations to furnish health care services;

    (5) The health maintenance organization is no longer financially responsible and may reasonably be expected to be unable to meet its obligations to enrollees or prospective enrollees;

    (6) The health maintenance organization has failed to correct, within the time prescribed by Subsection C, any deficiency occurring due to such health maintenance organization's prescribed minimum net worth being impaired;

    (7) The health maintenance organization has failed to implement the grievance procedures required by Section 11 in a reasonable manner to resolve valid complaints;

    (8) The health maintenance organization, or any person on its behalf, has advertised or

merchandised its services in an untrue, misrepresentative, misleading, deceptive or unfair manner;

(9) The continued operation of the health maintenance organization would be hazardous to its enrollees; or

(10) The health maintenance organization has otherwise failed substantially to comply with this Act.

B. In addition to or in lieu of suspension or revocation of a certificate of authority pursuant to this section, the applicant or health maintenance organization may be subjected to an administrative penalty of up to [insert amount] dollars for each cause for suspension or revocation.

C. The following shall pertain when insufficient net worth is maintained:

(1) Whenever the commissioner [director, superintendent] finds that the net worth maintained by any health maintenance organization subject to the provisions of this Act is less than the minimum net worth required to be maintained by Section 13 of this Act, he shall give written notice to the health maintenance organization of the amount of the deficiency and require: (a) filing with the commissioner [director, superintendent] a plan for correction of the deficiency acceptable to the commissioner [director, superintendent] and (b) correction of the deficiency within a reasonable time, not to exceed sixty (60) days, unless an extension of time, not to exceed sixty (60) additional days, is granted by the commissioner [director, superintendent]. Such a deficiency shall be deemed an impairment, and failure to correct the impairment in the prescribed time shall be grounds for suspension or revocation of the certificate of authority or for placing the health maintenance organization in conservation, rehabilitation or liquidation.

(2) Unless allowed by the commissioner [director, superintendent] no health maintenance organization or person acting on its behalf may, directly or indirectly, renew, issue or deliver any certificate, agreement or contract of coverage in this state, for which a premium is charged or collected, when the health maintenance organization writing such coverage is impaired, and the fact of such impairment is known to the health maintenance organization or to such person.

However, the existence of an impairment shall not prevent the issuance or renewal of a certificate, agreement or contract when the enrollee exercises an option granted under the plan to obtain a new, renewed or converted coverage.

D. A certificate of authority shall be suspended or revoked or an application or a certificate of authority denied or an administrative penalty imposed only after compliance with the requirements of this section.

(1) Suspension or revocation of a certificate of authority or the denial of an application or the imposition of an administrative penalty pursuant to this section shall be by written order and shall be sent to the health maintenance organization or applicant by certified or registered mail and to the [commissioner of public health]. The written order shall state the grounds, charges or conduct on which suspension, revoca-

tion or denial or administrative penalty is based. The health maintenance organization or applicant may in writing request a hearing within thirty (30) days from the date of mailing of the order. If no written request is made, such order shall be final upon the expiration of said thirty (30) days.

(2) If the health maintenance organization or applicant requests a hearing pursuant to this section, the commissioner [director, superintendent] shall issue a written notice of hearing and send it to the health maintenance organization or applicant by certified or registered mail and to the [commissioner of public health] stating:

(a) A specific time for the hearing, which may not be less than twenty (20) nor more than thirty (30) days after mailing of the notice of hearing; and

(b) A specific place for the hearing, which may be either in [location of regulatory body] or in the county where the health maintenance organization's or applicant's principal place of business is located.

(c) If a hearing is requested, the [commissioner of public health] or his designated representative shall be in attendance and shall participate in the proceedings. The recommendations and findings of the [commissioner of public health] with respect to matters relating to the quality of health care services provided in connection with any decision regarding denial, suspension or revocation of a certificate of authority, shall be conclusive and binding upon the commissioner [director, superintendent].

After such hearing, or upon failure of the health maintenance organization to appear at such hearing, the commissioner [director, superintendent] shall take whatever action he deems necessary based on written findings and shall mail his decision to the health maintenance organization or applicant with a copy to the [commissioner of public health]. The action of the commissioner [director, superintendent] and the recommendation and findings of the [commissioner of public health] shall be subject to review under the State Administrative Review Act (or other applicable statutory review process).

E. The provisions of the [Administrative Procedure Act] of this state shall apply to proceedings under this section to the extent they are not in conflict with Subsection D(2).

F. When the certificate of authority of a health maintenance organization is suspended, the health maintenance organization shall not, during the period of such suspension, enroll any additional enrollees except newborn children or other newly acquired dependents of existing enrollees, and shall not engage in any advertising or solicitation whatsoever.

G. When the certificate of authority of a health maintenance organization is revoked, such organization shall proceed, immediately following the effective date of the order of revocation, to wind up its affairs, and shall conduct no further business except as may be essential to the orderly conclusion of the affairs of such organization. It shall engage in no further advertising or solicitation whatsoever. The commissioner [director, superintendent] may, by written order, permit such further operation of the organization as he may find to be in the best interest of enrollees, to the end that enrollees will be afforded the greatest practical opportunity to obtain continuing health care coverage.

Section 21. Rehabilitation, Liquidation or Conservation of Health Maintenance Organizations

A. Any rehabilitation, liquidation or conservation of a health maintenance organization shall be deemed to be the rehabilitation, liquidation or conservation of an insurance company and shall be conducted under the supervision of the commissioner [director, superintendent] pursuant to the law governing the rehabilitation, liquidation or conservation of insurance companies. The commissioner [director, superintendent] may apply for an order directing him to rehabilitate, liquidate or conserve a health maintenance organization upon any one or more grounds set out in [cite sections of state rehabilitation law], or when in his opinion the continued operation of the health maintenance organization would be hazardous either to the enrollees or to the people of this state. Enrollees shall have the same priority in the event of liquidation or rehabilitation as the law provides to policyholders of an insurer.

B. For purpose of determining the priority of distribution of general assets, claims of enrollees and enrollees' beneficiaries shall have the same priority as established by [insert state statute for liquidation of insurers] for policyholders and beneficiaries of insureds of insurance companies. If an enrollee is liable to any provider for services provided pursuant to and covered by the health care plan, that liability shall have the status of an enrollee claim for distribution of general assets.

Any provider who is obligated by statute or agreement to hold enrollees harmless from liability for services provided pursuant to and covered by a health care plan shall have a priority of distribution of the general assets immediately following that of enrollees and enrollees' beneficiaries as described herein, and immediately preceding the priority of distribution described in [insert citation to insurance code].

Section 22. Summary Orders and Supervision

A. Whenever the commissioner [director, superintendent] determines that the financial condition of any health maintenance organization is such that its continued operation might be hazardous to its enrollees, creditors, or the general public, or that it has violated any provision of this Act, he may, after notice and hearing, order the health maintenance organization to take such action as may be reasonably necessary to rectify such condition or violation, including but not limited to one or more of the following:

(1) Reduce the total amount of present and potential liability for benefits by reinsurance or other method acceptable to the commissioner [director, superintendent];

(2) Reduce the volume of new business being accepted;

(3) Reduce expenses by specified methods;

(4) Suspend or limit the writing of new business for a period of time;

(5) Increase the health maintenance organization's capital and surplus by contribution; or

(6) Take such other steps as the commissioner [director, superintendent] may deem appropriate under the circumstances.

B. For purposes of this section, the violation by a health maintenance organization of any law of this state to which such health maintenance organization is subject shall be deemed a violation of this Act.

C. The commissioner [director, superintendent] is authorized, by rules and regulations, to set uniform standards and criteria for early warning that the continued operation of any health maintenance organization might be hazardous to its enrollees, creditors, or the general public and to set standards for evaluating the financial condition of any health maintenance organization, which standards shall be consistent with the purposes expressed in Subsection A of this section.

D. The remedies and measures available to the commissioner [director, superintendent] under this section shall be in addition to, and not in lieu of, the remedies and measures available to the commissioner [director, superintendent] under the provisions of [cite law which implements Sections 9 and 10 of the NAIC Rehabilitation and Liquidation Model Act].

Section 23. Regulations

The commissioner [director, superintendent] may, after notice and hearing, promulgate reasonable rules and regulations, as are necessary or proper to carry out the provisions of this Act. Such rules and regulations shall be subject to review in accordance with [insert statutory citation providing for administrative rulemaking and review of such rules].

Section 24. Fees

A. Every health maintenance organization subject to this Act shall pay to the commissioner [director, superintendent] the following fees:

(1) For filing an application for a certificate of authority or amendment thereto [insert amount] dollars;

(2) For filing an amendment to the organization documents that requires approval, [insert amount] dollars;

(3) For filing an amendment "for information only," [insert amount] dollars; and

(4) For filing each annual report, [insert amount] dollars.

B. Fees charged under this section shall be distributed as follows: [insert dollar amount] to the commissioner [director, superintendent] and [insert dollar amount] to the [commissioner of public health].

[Alternative language to Subsections A and B above:

The commissioner [director, superintendent] shall promulgate rules for collecting fees from health maintenance organizations.]

Comment: Each state should examine its statutory authority to collect fees and select the appropriate language suggested above.

Section 25. Penalties and Enforcement

A. The commissioner [director, superintendent] may, in lieu of suspension or revocation of a certificate of authority under Section 20, levy an administrative penalty in an amount not less than [insert amount] dollars nor more than [insert amount] dollars, if reasonable notice in writing is given of the intent to levy the penalty and the health maintenance organization has a reasonable time within which to remedy the defect in its operations which gave rise to the penalty citation. The commissioner [director, superintendent] may augment this penalty by an amount equal to the sum that he calculates to be the damages suffered by enrollees or other members of the public.

B. (1) If the commissioner [director, superintendent] or the [commissioner of public health] shall for any reason have cause to believe that any violation of this Act has occurred or is threatened, the commissioner [director, superintendent] or [commissioner of public health] may give notice to the health maintenance organization and to the representatives, or other persons who appear to be involved in such suspected violation, to arrange a conference with the alleged violators or their authorized representatives for the purpose of attempting to ascertain the facts relating to such suspected violation; and, in the event it appears that any violation has occurred or is threatened, to arrive at an adequate and effective means of correcting or preventing such violation.

(2) Proceedings under this subsection shall not be governed by any formal procedural requirements, and may be conducted in such manner as the commissioner [director, superintendent] or the [commissioner of public health] may deem appropriate under the circumstances. However, unless consented to by the health maintenance organization, no rule or order may result from a conference until the requirements of this section of this Act are satisfied.

C. (1) The commissioner [director, superintendent] may issue an order directing a health maintenance organization or a representative of a health maintenance organization to cease and desist from engaging in any act or practice in violation of the provisions of this Act.

(2) Within [insert number] days after service of the cease and desist order, the respondent may request a hearing on the question of whether acts or practices in violation of this Act have occurred. Such hearings shall be conducted pursuant to [cite sections of state administrative procedure act], and judicial review shall be available as provided by [cite sections of state administrative procedure act].

D. In the case of any violation of the provisions of this Act, if the commissioner [director, superintendent] elects not to issue a cease and desist order, or in the event of noncompliance with a cease and desist order issued pursuant to Subsection C, the commissioner [director, superintendent] may institute a proceeding to obtain injunctive or other appropriate relief in the [name of court of primary jurisdiction for actions of this nature].

Comment: Sections 25C and 25D authorize the commissioner to issue a cease and desist order and to apply for injunctive relief. When the commissioner is not granted such statutory powers, the language should be modified to provide for the legal steps to be taken by the attorney general or other appropriate state official.

E. Notwithstanding any other provisions of this Act, if a health maintenance organization fails to comply with the net worth requirement of this Act, the commissioner [director, superintendent] is authorized to take appropriate action to assure that the continued operation of the health maintenance organization will not be hazardous to its enrollees.

Section 26. Statutory Construction and Relationship to Other Laws

A. Except as otherwise provided in this Act, provisions of the insurance law and provisions of hospital or medical service corporation laws shall not be applicable to any health maintenance organization granted a certificate of authority under this Act. This provision shall not apply to an insurer or hospital or medical service corporation licensed and regulated pursuant to the insurance law or the hospital or medical service corporation laws of this state except with respect to its health maintenance organization activities authorized and regulated pursuant to this Act.

B. Solicitation of enrollees by a health maintenance organization granted a certificate of authority, or its representatives, shall not be construed to violate any provision of law relating to solicitation or advertising by health professionals.

C. Any health maintenance organization authorized under this Act shall not be deemed to be practicing medicine and shall be exempt from the provision of [citation] relating to the practice of medicine.

Section 27. Filings and Reports as Public Documents

All applications, filings and reports required under this Act shall be treated as public documents, except those which are trade secrets or privileged or confidential quality assurance, commercial or financial information, other than any annual financial statement that may be required under Section 9 of this Act.

Section 28. Confidentiality of Medical Information and Limitation of Liability

A. Any data or information pertaining to the diagnosis, treatment or health of any enrollee or applicant obtained from such person or from any provider by any health maintenance organization shall be held in confidence and shall not be disclosed to any person except to the extent that it may be necessary to carry out the purposes of this Act; or upon the express consent of the enrollee or applicant; or pursuant to statute or court order for the production of evidence or the discovery thereof; or in the event of claim or litigation between such person and the health maintenance organization wherein such data or information is pertinent. A health maintenance organization shall be entitled to claim any statutory privileges against such disclosure which the provider who furnished such information to the health maintenance organization is entitled to claim.

B. A person who, in good faith and without malice, takes any action or makes any decision or recommendation as a member, agent or employee of a health care review committee or who furnishes any records, information or assistance to such a committee shall not be subject to liability for civil damages or any legal action in consequence of such action, nor shall the health maintenance organization which established such committee or the officers, directors, employees or agents of such health maintenance organization be liable for the activities of any such person. This section shall not be construed to relieve any person of liability arising from treatment of a patient.

C. (1) The information considered by a health care review committee and the records of their actions and proceedings shall be confidential and not subject to subpoena or order to produce except in proceedings before the appropriate state licensing or certifying agency, or in an appeal, if permitted, from the committee's findings or recommendations. No member of a health care review committee, or officer, director or other member of a health maintenance organization or its staff engaged in assisting such committee, or any person assisting or furnishing information to such committee may be subpoenaed to testify in any judicial or quasi-judicial proceeding if such subpoena is based solely on such activities.

(2) Information considered by a health care review committee and the records of its actions and proceedings which are used pursuant to Subsection C(1) by a state licensing or certifying agency or in an appeal shall be kept confidential and shall be subject to the same provision concerning discovery and use in legal actions as are the original information and records in the possession and control of a health care review committee.

D. To fulfill its obligations under Section 7, the health maintenance organization shall have access to treatment records and other information pertaining to the diagnosis, treatment or health status of any enrollee.

Section 29. [Commissioner of Public Health's] Authority to Contract

The [commissioner of public health], in carrying out his obligations under this Act, may contract with qualified persons to make recommendations concerning the determinations required to be made by him. Such recommendations may be accepted in full or in part by the [commissioner of public health].

Section 30. Acquisition of Control of or Merger of a Health Maintenance Organization

No person may make a tender for or a request or invitation for tenders of, or enter into an agreement to exchange securities for or acquire in the open market or otherwise, any voting security of a health maintenance organization or enter into any other agreement if, after the consummation thereof, that person would, directly or indirectly, (or by conversion or by exercise of any right to acquire) be in control of the health maintenance organization, and no person may enter into an agreement to merge or consolidate with or otherwise to acquire control of a health maintenance organization, unless, at the time any offer, request or invitation is made or any agreement is entered into, or prior to the acquisition of the securities if no offer or agreement is involved, the person has filed with the commissioner [director, superintendent] and has sent to the health maintenance organization, information required by Section [cite Sections 2(b)(1), (2), (3), (4), (5), and (12) of the NAIC Model Insurance Holding Company System Regulatory Act] and the offer, request, invitation, agreement or acquisition has been approved by the commissioner [director, superintendent]. Approval by the commissioner [director, superintendent] shall be governed by Section [cite law which implements Section 3(d)(1) and (2) of the NAIC Model Insurance Holding Company System Regulatory Act].

Section 31. Dual Choice [optional]

Each employer, public or private, in this state which offers its employees a health benefit plan and employs not less than twenty-five (25) employees, and each employee benefit func in this state which offers its members any form of basic health benefit, shall make available to and inform its employees or members of the option to enroll in at least one group practice health maintenance organization and one other health maintenance organization holding a valid certificate of authority which provides basic health care services in the geographic areas in which a substantial number of such employees or members reside. Where there is a prevailing collective bargaining agreement, the selection of the health maintenance organization(s) to be made available to the employees shall be made under the agreement. No employer in this state shall be required to pay more for health benefits as a result of the application of this section than would otherwise be required by any prevailing collective bargaining agreement or other contract for the provision of basic health benefits to its employees. The employer or benefits fund shall pay to the health maintenance organization chosen by each employee or member an amount which does not financially discriminate against an employee who enrolls in such health maintenance organization. For purposes of the preceding sentence, an employer's contribution does not financially discriminate if the employer's method of determining the contributions on behalf of all employees is reasonable and is designed to assure employees a fair choice among health benefits plans.

Comment: This section, which is optional, is similar to Section 1310 of the federal Health Maintenance Organization Act, but extends the dual choice requirement to state licensed health maintenance organizations.

The purpose for this provision is to assist in the growth and development of state licensed health maintenance organizations. A state that wants to continue to promote the development of health maintenance organizations or to establish a standard on which employer contributions are made may want to enact this section.

Section 32. Coordination of Benefits

A. Health maintenance organizations are permitted, but not required, to adopt coordination of benefits provisions to avoid overinsurance and to provide for the orderly payment of claims when a person is covered by two or more group health insurance or health care plans.

B. If health maintenance organizations adopt coordination of benefits, the provisions must be consistent with the coordination of benefits provisions that are in general use in the state for coordinating coverage between two or more group health insurance or health care plans.

C. To the extent necessary for health maintenance organizations to meet their obligations as secondary carriers under the rules for coordination, health maintenance organizations shall make payments for services that are: received from non-participating providers; provided outside their service areas; or not covered under the terms of their group contracts or evidence of coverage.

Section 33. Insolvency Protection; Assessment

A. When a health maintenance organization in this state is declared insolvent by a court of competent jurisdiction, the commissioner [director, superintendent] may levy an assessment on health maintenance organizations doing business in this state to pay claims for uncovered expenditures for enrollees who are residents of this state and to provide continuation of coverage for subscribers or enrollees not covered under Section 15. The commissioner [director, superintendent] may not assess in any one calendar year more than two percent (2%) of the aggregate premium written by each health maintenance organization in this state the prior calendar year.

B. The commissioner [director, superintendent] may use funds obtained under Subsection A to pay claims for uncovered expenditures for subscribers or enrollees of an insolvent health maintenance organization who are residents of this state, provide for continuation of coverage for subscribers or enrollees who are residents of this state and are not covered under Section 15, and administrative costs. The commissioner [director, superintendent] may by regulation prescribe the time, manner and form for filing claims under this section or may require claims to be allowed by an ancillary receiver or the domestic liquidator or receiver.

C. (1) A receiver or liquidator of an insolvent health maintenance organization shall allow a claim in the proceeding in an amount equal to administrative and uncovered expenditures paid under this section.

    (2) Any person receiving benefits under this section for uncovered expenditures is deemed to have assigned the rights under the covered health care plan certificates to the commissioner [director, superintendent] to the extent of the benefits received. The commissioner [director, superintendent] may require an assignment to it of such rights by any payee, enrollee, or beneficiary as a condition precedent to the receipt of any rights or benefits conferred by this section upon such person. The commissioner [director, superintendent] is subrogated to these rights against the assets of any insolvent health maintenance organization held by a receiver or liquidator of another jurisdiction.

(3) The assignment or subrogation rights of the commissioner [director, superintendent] and allowed claim under this subsection have the same priority against the assets of the insolvent health maintenance organization as those possessed by the person entitled to receive benefits under this section or for similar expenses in the receivership or liquidation.

D. When assessed funds are unused following the completion of the liquidation of a health maintenance organization, the commissioner [director, superintendent] will distribute on a pro rata basis any amounts received under Subsection A which are not de minimis to the health maintenance organizations which have been assessed under this section.

E. The aggregate coverage of uncovered expenditures under this section shall not exceed $300,000 with respect to any one individual. Continuation of coverage shall not continue for more than the lesser of one year after the health maintenance organization coverage is terminated by insolvency or the remaining term of the contract. The commissioner [director, superintendent] may provide continuation of coverage on any reasonable basis, including but not limited to, continuation of the health maintenance organization contract or substitution of indemnity coverage in a form determined by the commissioner [director, superintendent].

F. The commissioner [director, superintendent] may waive an assessment of any health maintenance organization if it would be or is impaired or placed in financially hazardous condition. A health maintenance organization which fails to pay an assessment within thirty (30) days after notice is subject to a civil forfeiture of not more than $1,000 per day and/or suspension or revocation of its certificate of authority. Any action taken by the commissioner [director, superintendent] in enforcing the provisions of this section may be appealed by the health maintenance organization in accordance with [the administrative procedure act].

Drafting Comment: Section 33 is not recommended for all states. A state should carefully review its health maintenance organization market to determine whether the assessment procedure under this section is feasible. If health maintenance organization premium volume is small or dominated by a few organizations, a state may wish to rely solely on the protections provided under Section 14 and 15.

For those states where an assessment is feasible, this section provides assurance that funds will be available to pay uncovered expenditures even if those liabilities have been underestimated by the organization or have significantly escalated as the financial condition of the organization deteriorated. In addition, an assessment provides a means for continued coverage for those subscribers or enrollees who are not protected under Section 15.

Section 34. Severability

If any section, term, or provision of this Act shall be adjudged invalid for any reason, such judgment shall not affect, impair or invalidate any other section, term or provision of this Act; but the remaining sections, terms and provisions shall be and remain in full force and effect.

Legislative History (all references are to the *Proceedings of the NAIC*).

1973 Proc. I 9, 11, 141, 192, 202–222 (adopted).

1973 Proc. II 139 (synopsis of model).

1974 Proc. I 12, 14, 405, 413 (amended).

1982 Proc. I 19, 28, 431, 498–499, 530–554 (revised and reprinted).

1989 Proc. I 9, 22, 180–181, 327, 331–335 (amended).

1989 Proc. II 13, 25–26, 40, 51–79 (amended and reprinted).

1990 Proc. I 6, 26, 171, 374–376, 377–379 (amended).

1991 Proc. I (technical amendment).

Appendix C

PREFERRED PROVIDER ARRANGEMENTS MODEL ACT

Reprinted with the permission of the National Association of Insurance Commissioners (NAIC)

Table of Contents

Section 1. Short Title
Section 2. Purpose
Section 3. Definitions
Section 4. Preferred Provider Arrangements
Section 5. Health Benefit Plans
Section 6. Preferred Provider Participation Requirements
Section 7. General Requirements
Section 8. Regulations
Section 9. Severability

Section 1. Short Title

This Act shall be known and may be cited as the Preferred Provider Arrangements Act.

Section 2. Purpose

The purpose of this Act is to encourage health care cost containment while preserving quality of care by allowing health care insurers to enter into preferred provider arrangements and by establishing minimum standards for preferred provider arrangements and the health benefit plans associated with those arrangements.

Drafting Note: The use of the term "allowing" in this section is not intended to indicate that health care insurers are acting unlawfully in a state which has not enacted a law allowing Preferred Provider Arrangements.

Section 3. Definitions

The following words and phrases when used in this Act shall have the meanings given to them in this section unless the context clearly indicates otherwise:

A. Commissioner—The Insurance Commissioner of the State of ___________.

B. Covered Person—Any person on whose behalf the health care insurer is obligated to pay for or provide health care services.

C. Covered Services—Health care services which the health care insurer is obligated to pay for or provide under the Health Benefit Plan.

D. Emergency Care—Covered services delivered to a covered person who has suffered an accidental bodily injury or contracted a medical condition which reasonably requires the beneficiary or insured to seek immediate medical care under circumstances or at locations which reasonably preclude the beneficiary or insured from obtaining needed medical care from a preferred provider.

E. Health Benefit Plan—The health insurance policy or subscriber agreement between the covered person or the policyholder and the health care insurer which defines the covered services and benefit levels available.

F. Health Care Insurer—An insurance company as defined in _____________, a hospital plan corporation as defined in _____________, a health services plan corporation as defined in _____________, a health maintenance organization as defined in _____________, or a fraternal benefit society as defined in _____________.

Drafting Note: This definition may need to be modified to conform to the state's service plan enabling statutes.

G. Health Care Provider—Providers of health care services licensed as required in this State.

H. Health Care Services—Services rendered or products sold by a health care provider within the scope of the provider's license. The term includes, but is not limited to, hospital, medical, surgical, dental, vision, and pharmaceutical services or products.

I. Preferred Provider—A health care provider or group of providers who have contracted to provide specified covered services.

J. Preferred Provider Arrangement—A contract between or on behalf of the health care insurer and a preferred provider which complies with all the requirements of this Act.

Section 4. Preferred Provider Arrangements

Notwithstanding any provisions of law to the contrary, any health care insurer may enter into Preferred Provider Arrangements.

A. Such arrangements shall:

(1) Establish the amount and manner of payment to the preferred provider. Such amount and manner of payment may include capitation payments for preferred providers.

(2) Include mechanisms which are designed to minimize the cost of the health benefit plan. These mechanisms may include among others:

(a) The review or control of utilization of health care services.

(b) A procedure for determining whether health care services rendered are medically necessary.

(3) Assure reasonable access to covered services available under the Preferred Provider Arrangement and an adequate number of preferred providers to render those services.

B. Such arrangements shall not unfairly deny health benefits for medically necessary covered services.

C. If an entity enters into a contract providing covered services with a health care provider, but is not engaged in activities which would require it to be licensed as a health care insurer, such entity shall file with the Insurance Commissioner information describing its activities and a description of the contract or agreement it has entered into with the health care providers. Employers who enter into contracts with health care providers for the exclusive benefit of their employees and dependents are exempt from this requirement.

Drafting Note: Section 4C is an optional section if a state desires to require verification of PPO activity of non-insurance entities.

Section 5. Health Benefit Plans

A. Health care insurers may issue health benefit plans which provide for incentives for covered persons to use the health care services of preferred providers. Such policies or subscriber agreements shall contain at least the following provisions:

(1) A provision that if a covered person receives emergency care for services specified in the Preferred Provider Arrangement and cannot reasonably reach a preferred provider that emergency care rendered during the course of the emergency will be reimbursed as though the covered person had been treated by a preferred provider; and

(2) A provision which clearly identifies the differentials in benefit levels for health care services of preferred providers and benefit levels for health care services of non-preferred providers.

B. If a health benefit plan provides differences in benefit levels payable to preferred providers compared to other providers, such differences shall not unfairly deny payment for covered services and shall be no greater than necessary to provide a reasonable incentive for covered persons to use the preferred provider.

Section 6. Preferred Provider Participation Requirements

Health care insurers may place reasonable limits on the number or classes of preferred providers which satisfy the standards set forth by the health care insurer, provided that there be no discrimination against providers on the basis of religion, race, color, national origin, age, sex or marital status, and further provided that selection of preferred providers is primarily based on, but not limited to, cost and availability of covered services and the quality of services performed by the providers.

Drafting Notes: Categories of Discrimination—Individual states may wish to add additional protected classes in accordance with state laws or policies.

Quality of Services—The statement of a quality criterion as used in this section is not intended to create any higher standard of care for delivery of services by a preferred provider than is appropriate for other health care providers.

Section 7. General Requirements

Health care insurers complying with this Act shall be subject to and are required to comply with all other applicable laws, rules and regulations of this State.

Section 8. Regulations

The Commissioner may promulgate regulations necessary to the enforcement and administration of this Act.

Section 9. Severability

If any provision of this Act is declared invalid or unenforceable by a court of competent jurisdiction, the remaining provisions which are severable from the invalid provisions shall remain in force and effect.

Drafting Note: If a state elects to permit exclusive provider arrangements, the following section should be added to the Act:

Notwithstanding any other provision of this Act, health care insurers may issue policies or subscriber agreements which provide benefits for health care services only if the services have been rendered by a preferred provider, provided the program has met all standards imposed by the Commissioner for availability and adequacy of covered services.

Legislative History (all references are to the *Proceedings of the NAIC*).

1987 Proc. I 11, 19, 652, 713, 716–718 (adopted).

NOTES

1. Matthew D. Rifkin, M.D., et al., "Comparison of Magnetic Resonance Imaging and Ultrasonography in Staging Early Prostate Cancer: Results of a Multi-Institutional Cooperative Trial," *The New England Journal of Medicine* (September 6, 1990), 626. *See also* Bernard G. Ewigman, M.D., et al., "Effect of Prenatal Ultrasound Screening on Perinatal Outcome," *The New England Journal of Medicine* (September 16, 1993), 826; P.S. Conti, J.S. Keppler, and J.M. Halls, "Positron Emission Tomography: A Financial and Operational Analysis," *American Journal of Roentgenology* (Los Angeles: University of Southern California, June 1994), 1279–86; B.J. Hillman, "New Imaging Technology and Cost Containment," *American Journal of Roentgenology* (Charlottesville, Virginia: University of Virginia School of Medicine and Health Sciences Center, March 1994), 503–6.

2. Victor R. Fuchs, *Who Shall Live? Health Economics and Social Choice* (New York: Basic Books, Inc., 1974), 54–55.

3. The Wyatt Company, *Report to the Health Insurance Association of America: Cost Analysis of State Legislative Mandates on Six Managed Health Care Practices* (June 7, 1991), 15–20.

4. Jon Gabel and Gail Jensen, "The Price of State Mandated Benefits," *Research Bulletin* (Washington, D.C.: HIAA, July 1989), 17.

5. Physician Payment Review Commission, *Annual Report to Congress* (Washington, D.C., 1994), 9.

6. Ibid., 13–14.

7. 1994 Green Book: Background Material and Data on Programs within the Jurisdiction of the Committee on Ways and Means (Washington, D.C.: US Government Printing Office, 1994), 854.

8. M. Mitka, "Government Report: Is Medicare HMO Cost Effective?" *American Medical News* (October 10, 1994), 4.

9. Deborah H. Harrison and John R. Kimberly, "HMOs Don't Have to Fail," *Harvard Business Review,* Volume 60 (July–August 1982), 115–124.

10. Lynn R. Gruber, Maureen Shadle, and Cynthia C. Polich, "From Movement to Industry: The Growth of HMOs," *Health Affairs,* Volume 1.7, No. 3 (Summer 1988), 198.

11. *Source Book of Health Insurance Data* (Washington, D.C.: HIAA, 1994).

12. Elizabeth Hoy, *Insurer-Sponsored Managed Health Care 1990* (Washington, D.C.: HIAA, 1991), 5.

13. Hoy, 5.

14. Judy Packer-Tursman, "Blues Policy Shifts to MCOs," *Managed Health Care News,* Volume 2, No. 8 (August 17, 1992), 32.

15. Anthony R. Masso and Wendy Knight Haesler, "The Impact of Managed Care on the Health Insurance Industry," *Journal of Insurance Medicine,* Volume 23, No. 3 (Fall 1991), 155.

16. Cynthia B. Sullivan, Ph.D., Marianne Miller, M.A. and Claudia C. Johnson, M.P.H., M.P.P., *Employer-Sponsored Health Insurance in 1991* (Washington, D.C.: HIAA, 1992), 7-8.

17. Group Health Association of America, *National Directory of HMOs* (Washington, D.C.: GHAA, 1991), 19.

18. HIAA Employer Survey, 1992.

19. American Hospital Association, *State of the Art of Managed Care 1993-1994: A Special Report by the Healthcare Provider Network Section of the Society of Healthcare Planning and Marketing* (Chicago: AHA, 1993). *See also* Emmons and Simon, *Recent Trends in Managed Care* (Chicago: AMA, 1994).

20. Sharon George-Perry, "Easing the Costs of Mental Health Benefits," *Personnel Administrator,* Volume 33 (November 1988), 62-67.

21. Employee Benefit Research Institute, "Prescription Drugs: Coverage, Costs and Quality," EBRI Issue Brief No. 122 (Washington, D.C.: EBRI, January 1992)

22. United States Senate, Special Committee on Aging, "The Drug Manufacturing Industry: Prescription for Profits 1980-1990," 102d Congress, 1st Session September 1991.

23. United States General Accounting Office, "Prescription Drugs: Changes in Prices for Selected Drugs," GAO/HRD-92-128 (Washington, D.C.: GAO, August 1992).

24. *National Directory of HMOs* (1994), 27.

25. Interstudy, *The Interstudy Competitive Edge,* Volume 2, No. 1 (Excelsior, Minn.: InterStudy, 1991), 14.

26. *National Directory of HMOs* (1994), 27.

27. *National Directory of HMOs* (1994), 27.

28. Nancy Kraus, Michelle Porter, and Patricia Ball, *Managed Care: A Decade in Review 1980-1990, The InterStudy Edge* (1991), 79. *See also National Directory of HMOs* (1994), 27.

29. National Rural Electric Cooperative Association and the Metropolitan Life Insurance Company, "Managed Care Plans in Rural America," (Washington, D.C.: National Rural Electric Cooperative Association, 1991), 6-10.

30. Marianne Miller and Thomas H. Dial, *Employer-Sponsored Health Insurance In Private Sector Firms in 1992* (Washington, D.C.: HIAA, 1993), 10.

31. Ibid.

32. Jon Gabel, et al., *Research Bulletin—The Health Insurance Picture in 1988* (Washington, D.C.: HIAA, July 1989), 3, 7, 11, 12.

33. Miller and Dial, 10.

34. "The Effects of Managed Care on the Use and Costs of Health Services," United States Congress, U.S. House of Representatives, Congressional Budget Office (Washington, D.C., June 1992), 8.

35. Jon Gabel and Derek Liston, *Trends in Health Insurance—HMOs Experience Lower Rates of Increase than Other Plans* (Washington, D.C.: KPMG Peat Marwick, December 1993), 14.

36. Fuchs, 54–55.

37. The Gallup Organization, Inc., "The Satisfaction Level of Managed Health Care Members Compared with Members of Indemnity Insurance Programs," a national poll (Princeton, N.J.: Gallup, 1991).

38. Towers Perrin, "Managed Care: The Employee Perspective," (New York: Towers Perrin, 1991).

39. A. Foster Higgins, Inc., "The Public Sector: City and State Governments," *Health Care Benefits Survey* (Princeton, N.J.: A. Foster Higgins, Inc., 1991), 1.

40. HIAA Employer Survey, 1992.

41. A. Foster Higgins, Inc., *Health Care Benefits Survey, Report 1, Indemnity Plans, Cost, Design, and Funding* (Princeton, N.J.: A. Foster Higgins, Inc., 1991), 14.

42. Clare Lippert and Eliott Wicks, *Critical Distinctions: How Firms That Offer Health Benefits Differ From Those That Do Not* (Washington, D.C.: HIAA, 1991), 4.

43. HIAA Employer Survey, 1990.

44. Metropolitan Life Insurance Company, "Trade Offs & Choices: Health Policy Options for the 1990s," a survey by Louis Harris & Associates (New York, 1991), 61.

45. The Wyatt Company, *A Cost Analysis of Three State Mandates to Regulate the Provision of Prescription Drug Benefits* (Washington, D.C.: The Wyatt Company, June 1992).

46. Mitka, 4.

47. E. Sholdice, *Introduction to Managed Care* (Arlington, VA: Information Resources Press, 1991), 136.

48. Information from the Group Health Association of America, as reported by the Bureau of National Affairs, "Medicare, Medicaid Contract Experience Eating into Plan's Commercial Business," BNA Medicare Report, Volume 2, No. 4, 182-183.

49. Mitka, 4.

50. United States General Accounting Office, "Health Insurance for the Elderly, Owning Duplicate Policies Is Costly and Unnecessary," *Report to Congressional Requestors* (Washington, D.C., 1994), 7.

51. Daniel R. Waldo, et al., "Health Expenditures by Age Group, 1977 and 1987," *Health Care Financing Review* (Baltimore, Maryland: U.S. Department of Health and Human Services, August 1989), 111.

52. Shelda L. Harden, *What Legislators Need To Know About Managed Care* (Washington, D.C.: National Conference of State Legislatures, 1994), 9.

53. Information from HCFA as reported to the Health Insurance Association of America; data appear in "Medicaid Programs Introduce Managed Care to Enhance Quality and Cost Containment," unpublished article, 1992.

54. Harry C. Schnibbe and E. Clarke Ross, "Moynihan Modifies Medicaid Managed Care Bill," *NASMHPD Report: The U.S. Congress, no. 102-54* (August 29, 1992), 2.

55. "Medicaid Waivers: More Flex in State Health Care 'Muscle,'" summary of proceedings from a concurrent session at the 17th Annual Meeting, National Conference of State Legislatures, Denver, Colorado, and Orlando, Florida, August 15, 1991.

56. Ibid.

57. Judith Miller Jones and Jack Hoadley, "Medicaid Managed Care: Is There Hope for This Marriage," *Issue Brief, No. 573* (Washington, D.C.: The George Washington University, 1991), 7-8.

58. John F. Boyer, David J. Fant and Chris J. Pool, "An Overview of Managed Health Care in the Department of Defense," *Medical Interface*, Volume 4, No. 11 (November 1991), 15-22.

59. J. Creedon et al., *Report on Federal Employees Health Benefits Program*, 102d Congress, U.S. House of Representatives, Committee on Post Office and Civil Service, Serial No. 102-6 (May 1992), 6.

60. Creedon, et al., 20.

61. Creedon, et al., 23. *See also* Towers Perrin, Forster and Crosby, *The Federal Employees Health Benefits Program* (Washington, D.C.: U.S. Office of Personnel Management, April 1988), 120.

62. 1992 Survey of State Employee Health Benefit Plans, (New York, N.Y.: The Segal Company, March 1992), 8-9.

63. The Martin Segal Company, 43–47.

64. HIAA, "Managed Care Facts," *Managed Care Bulletin* (February 1992), 3–4.

65. Brenda Trolin, "Workers' Compensation: 24 Hour Coverage," *NCSL LegisBrief* 1, no. 8 (February 1993), 1.

66. Keith T. Bateman and Cynthia J. Veldman, "24 Hour Coverage: An Analysis and Report about Current Developments," *Workers' Compensation Insurance Issues* (Schaumburg, Illinois: Alliance of American Insurers, February 1991), i, ii.

67. Sophie M. Koorczyk and Hazel A. Witte, *The NRECA Report on Managed Care Plans in Rural America: How They Work, What They Do* (Washington, D.C.: The National Rural Electric Cooperative Association and the Metropolitan Life Insurance Company, September 1991), 4.

68. Interim Task Force on State Welfare and Medicaid Reform, *Initial Recommendations for a Medicaid Managed Care Program* (October 29, 1992), 2.

69. S. Bernstein and L. Hilborne, "Clinical Indicators: The Road to Quality Care?" *Journal on Quality Care* (1993) 19(11), 501.

70. M. Ballard and J. Terze, "Automated Credentialling: A Practical Approach to Quality Management," *AAPPO Journal* (June/July 1993), 10–13.

71. J. Williamson and Associates, "Teaching Quality Assurance and Cost Containment in Health Care," *Association of Medical Colleges Series in Academic Medicine* (Washington, DC: Jossey-Bass Publishers, 1982).

72. W.E. Demings, *Out of Crisis* (Boston: Massachusetts Institute of Technology, 1986).

73. Hospital Corporation of America, "Hospital Wide Quality Improvement Process, Strategy for Improvement, FOCUS-PDCA" (Nashville, TN: Hospital Corporation of America, 1989).

74. E. Zablocki, "Getting Accurate Data in Sufficient Quantities is Only the First Step," *HMO* (November/December 1992), 32–36.

75. E. Pascuzzi, "Claims and Benefits Administration," *The Managed Health Care Handbook,* second edition (Gaithersburg, MD: Aspen Publishers, 1993), 211–230.

76. Pascuzzi, 211–230.

77. NCQA, HEDIS 2.0 Executive Summary (Washington, DC: NCQA, 1993).

GLOSSARY

A

ACCESS   Right to enter or use health care services.

ADJUSTED AVERAGE PER CAPITA COST (AAPCC)   Health Care Financing Administration (HCFA) basis of payment to HMOs and CMPs.

ADJUSTED COMMUNITY RATE (ACR)   Uniform capitation rate charged to all enrollees in a plan based on adjustments for risk factors such as age and sex.

AID TO FAMILIES WITH DEPENDENT CHILDREN (AFDC)   Public assistance program of social payments to families with children 18 years of age and under who have income below a defined poverty line.

AMBULATORY CARE   Medical services provided on an outpatient (nonhospitalized) basis. Services may include diagnosis, treatment, surgery, and rehabilitation.

ANCILLARY SERVICES   Health care services conducted by providers other than primary care physicians.

ANNUAL BENEFIT CAP   Maximum dollar amount paid for specific medical services.

AUTHORIZATIONS   Consent or endorsement by a primary care physician for patient referral to ancillary services and specialists.

AVERAGE LENGTH OF STAY   One measure of use of health facilities, reported as an average number of inpatient days spent in a hospital or other health care facility per admission or discharge. It is calculated as follows: total number of days in the facility for all admissions occurring during a period divided by the number of admissions during the same period. Average lengths of stay vary and are measured for patients based upon age, specific diagnoses, or sources of payment.

B

BALANCE BILLING   Practice by providers of billing patients for all charges over the physician rate paid by insurers. Many managed care plans prohibit the use of balance billing and may use sanctions against providers who balance bill.

BENCHMARK   Point of comparison between desired clinical outcome and actual practice.

BENEFIT   Amount payable by an insurance company to a claimant, assignee, or beneficiary when the insured suffers a loss covered by the policy.

C

CAPITATION   Method of payment for health services in which a physician or hospital is paid a fixed amount for each enrollee regardless of the actual number or nature of services provided to each person.

CARVE-OUT   Term used to describe certain services not included in capitated benefits that are paid for separately on a predetermined fee-for-service basis.

CASE MANAGEMENT   Planned approach to manage service or treatment to an individual with a serious medical problem. Its dual goal is to contain costs and promote more effective intervention to meet patient needs. Often referred to as large case management.

CIVILIAN HEALTH AND MEDICAL PROGRAM OF THE UNIFORMED SERVICES (CHAMPUS)   Federal program providing cost-sharing health benefits for dependents and survivors of active duty personnel and for retirees and their dependents and survivors.

CLAIM   Demand to the insurer by or on behalf of an insured person for the payment of benefits under a policy.

CLOSED PANEL   Managed care plan that contracts with physicians on an exclusive basis to provide health services to enrollees. Nonplan physicians are excluded from participation.

COINSURANCE   Portion of incurred medical expenses, usually a fixed percentage, that the patient must pay out of pocket. Also referred to as copayment.

COMMUNITY-RATED   Method of developing group-specific capitation rates by a health plan that generally does not account for unique characteristics of the group. The rate is based on the total experience of a given geographic area or "community."

COMPETITIVE MEDICAL PLANS (CMPS)   Health care organization that meets specific government criteria for Medicare risk contracting but is not necessarily a HMO.

CONCURRENT REVIEW   Method of utilization review that takes place on-site when a patient is confined to a hospital.

COORDINATION OF BENEFITS (COB)   Method of integrating benefits payable under more than one health insurance plan so that the insured's benefits from all sources do not exceed allowable medical expenses or eliminate appropriate patient incentives to contain costs.

COPAYMENT   See Coinsurance

COST SHIFTING   Transfer of health care provider costs that are not adequately reimbursed by one payor to other payors.

CREDENTIALING   Review and documentation of professional providers including licensure, malpractice history, analysis of practice patterns, and certification.

CURRENT PROCEDURAL TERMINOLOGY (CPT)   Set of five-digit codes describing medical services delivered that are used for billing by professional providers.

CUSTOMER   Users of health care services, such as patients getting care or providers getting support services from laboratories; payers of service, such as individuals, employers, or the government; or the general public as beneficiaries of services.

D

DEDUCTIBLE   Amount of covered expenses that must be incurred and paid by an insured person before benefits become payable by the insurer.

DEFENSIVE MEDICINE   Extensive use of laboratory tests, increased hospital admissions, and extended hospital stays for the principal purpose of reducing the possibility of malpractice suits by patients or providing a good legal defense in the event of such lawsuits.

DIAGNOSIS-RELATED GROUPS (DRGs)   System of determining specific reimbursement fees based on the medical diagnosis of a patient.

DISCHARGE PLANNING   Assessment of an inpatient's medical condition for the purpose of arranging for appropriate continuing care upon leaving the facility. This planning includes how long the patient will be in the hospital, the expected outcome, and whether there are special needs or requirements on discharge.

E

ENROLLEE   Health plan participant, member, or eligible individual in a managed care program.

EXCLUSIVE PROVIDER ORGANIZATION (EPO)   Arrangement consisting of a group of providers who have a contract with an insurer, employer, third-party administrator, or other sponsoring group. Criteria for provider participation may be the same as those in PPOs but have a more restrictive provider selection and credentialing process.

EXPERIENCE-RATED   Determination of premium or capitation rates for a group risk based wholly or partly on that group's previous cost and utilization experience.

F

FEDERALLY QUALIFIED   Voluntary federal certification for HMOs.

FEE-FOR-SERVICE   Method of payment for provider services based on each visit or service rendered.

FEE SCHEDULE   Maximum dollar or unit allowances for health services that apply under a specific contract.

FORMULARY   List of preferred pharmaceutical products to be used by a managed care plan's network physicians. Formularies are based on evaluations of the efficacy, safety, and cost-effectiveness of drugs.

FREESTANDING PLAN   Unbundled or separate health care benefits apart from the basic health care plan, usually dental or vision care. Employees are allowed either to select the separate benefit or decline it for other alternatives. This choice of freestanding plans is often referred to as "cafeteria-type" benefits.

G

GATEKEEPER   Role description of the primary care physician in HMOs who serves to control utilization and referral of enrollees.

GLOBAL FEES   Negotiated fees that are all-inclusive (one fee is paid for the entire range of services provided for a specific episode or episodes of care).

GROUP-MODEL HMO   HMO staffing that occurs through contracting with multispeciality medical groups to care for plan members. Physicians are not employees of the HMO but are considered as a closed panel.

H

HEALTH CARE FINANCING ADMINISTRATION (HCFA)   Branch of the U.S Department of Health and Human Services charged with oversight and financial management of government-related health care programs such as Medicare and Medicaid.

HEALTH CARE PREPAYMENT PLAN (HCPP)   HCFA program allowing managed care groups that organize, finance, and deliver Medicare Part B services to be reimbursed for such services on a reasonable cost basis.

HEALTH MAINTENANCE ORGANIZATION (HMO)   Organization that provides for a wide range of comprehensive health care services for a specified group of enrollees for a fixed, periodic prepayment. There are several models of HMOs including the staff model, group model, independent practice association, and mixed model.

HOME HEALTH SERVICES   Comprehensive, medically necessary range of health services provided by a recognized provider organization to a patient in the home.

HOSPICE   Concept of care provided to terminally ill patients and their families that emphasizes emotional needs and coping with pain and death rather than cure.

HOSPITAL BILL AUDIT   Independent examination of hospital bills by a third party to determine if services and supplies charged to the patient were actually delivered and if the price charged was correct.

I

INDEMNITY INSURANCE   Health care insurance plan providing benefits in a predetermined amount for covered services. Traditionally, payment is made on a fee-for-service basis with no involvement by the insurer in the actual delivery of health care services.

INDIVIDUAL OR INDEPENDENT PRACTICE ASSOCIATION (IPA)   Association of individual physicians that provides services on a negotiated per capita rate, flat retainer fee, or negotiated fee-for-service basis. It is one model of HMO managed care.

INTEGRATED COVERAGE   Combinations of HMOs, indemnity plans, or PPOs into one health care plan.

J

JOINT COMMISSION ON ACCREDITATION OF HEALTHCARE ORGANIZATIONS (JCAHO)   Private, voluntary accrediting organization for all types of health care organizations. Its focus is the outcome, process, and excellence in health care.

L

LONG-TERM CARE   Continuum of maintenance, custodial, and health services to the chronically ill, disabled, or mentally impaired. Services may be provided on an inpatient basis (subacute care, rehabilitation facility, nursing home, mental hospital), outpatient, or at-home basis.

M

MALPRACTICE   Unprofessional, incompetent, or inappropriate medical care.

MANAGED CARE   Term used to describe the coordination of financing and provision of health care to produce high-quality health care for the lowest possible cost.

MANAGED INDEMNITY   Use of utilization controls in traditional fee-for-service health insurance plans in order to reduce cost and inappropriate care.

MANAGEMENT INFORMATION SYSTEMS (MIS)   Term used to describe computer systems that gather, store, and report information as needed. The three most common types are applications reporting systems, database management systems, and decision support systems.

MANDATED BENEFITS   Health care coverage required by state law to be included in health insurance contracts.

MEDICAID   State programs with federal matching funds for public health assistance to persons, regardless of age, whose income and resources are insufficient to pay for health care.

MEDICAL NECESSITY   Term use by insurers to describe medical treatment that is appropriate and rendered in accordance with generally accepted standards of medical practice.

MEDICARE   Federally sponsored program under the Social Security Act that provides hospital benefits, supplementary medical care, and catastrophic coverage to persons 65 years of age and older and some younger persons who are covered under Social Security benefits.

MEDICARE PART A   One of two parts of Medicare that pays for hospital services.

MEDICARE PART B   Voluntary part of Medicare that pays a percentage of reasonable and customary costs for physician and ancillary services.

MEDICARE-QUALIFIED PROVIDERS   Those providers who have been approved to receive payment for covered Medicare Part B.

MEDICARE RISK CONTRACT   Federal Medicare contract with HMOs or CMPs that pays a prospective monthly capitation payment for each Medicare member in the plan. The capitation payment is figured at an adjusted annual per capita cost (AAPCC) at no more than 95 percent of projected rates.

MEDICARE SELECT   Federal program designed to introduce Medicare beneficiaries to managed care systems through Preferred Provider Organization supplemental (MedSup) health insurance.

MENTAL HEALTH SERVICES   Behavioral health care services that may be provided on an inpatient, outpatient, or partial hospitalization basis.

MILITARY HEALTH SERVICES SYSTEM (MHSS)   Federal health benefits program for active duty military personnel, retirees, their dependents, and survivors.

MULTIPLE PROVIDER ARRANGEMENT   Managed care plan consisting of group, staff, or IPA structures in combination.

MULTISPECIALTY GROUP PRACTICE   Independent physicians' group that organizes or is organized to contract with a managed care plan to provide medical services to enrollees. The physicians are not employees of the HMO, but are employed by the group practice.

N

NATIONAL ASSOCIATION OF INSURANCE COMMISSIONERS (NAIC)   National organization of state officials charged with regulating insurance. It has no official power but wields tremendous influence. The association was formed to promote national uniformity in insurance regulations.

NATIONAL COMMITTEE ON QUALITY ASSURANCE (NCQA)   Private, voluntary accrediting organization for managed care. It assesses quality, credentialing, utilization management, customer rights, preventive health services, and medical records. Developer of the Health Plan Employer Data Set (HEDIS).

NEGOTIATED FEES   Managed care plans and providers mutually agree on a set fee for each service. This negotiated rate is usually based on services defined by the Current Procedural Terminology (CPT) codes, generally at a discount from what the provider would usually charge. Providers cannot charge more than this fee.

NETWORK OR MIXED-MODEL HMO   Provider arrangements that contract with a number of Independent Practice Associations or group practices to provide physician services to HMO enrollees. This model is a multiple provider arrangement that can be either an open or closed panel.

NETWORK PROVIDERS   Limited grouping or panel of providers in a managed care arrangement with several delivery points. Enrollees may be required to use only network providers or may have financing liability for using non-network providers for medical services.

NON-NETWORK PROVIDERS   Noncontracted or unapproved health providers who are outside a managed care arrangement.

O

OMNIBUS BUDGET RECONCILIATION ACT (OBRA)   Term given by Congress to many of its annual tax and budget reconciliation acts. Most of these tax and budget acts have language or provisions related to health care and managed care, particularly in relation to Medicare services.

OPEN-ENDED HMO   Hybrid HMO product that allows members to use physicians outside the plan in exchange for additional personal liability in the form of a deductible, coinsurance, or copayment.

OUTCOME MEASUREMENT   Tool used to assess a health system's performance that measures the outcome of a given intervention.

OUT-OF-NETWORK CARE   Medical services obtained by managed care plan members from unaffiliated or noncontracted health care providers. In many plans, such care will not be reimbursed unless previous authorization for such care is obtained.

OUT-OF-POCKET EXPENSES   Those health care costs that must be borne by the insured because they are not covered under an insurance contract.

OVERUTILIZATION   Term used to describe inappropriate or excessive use of medical services that add to health care costs.

P

PARTIAL CAPITATION RISK CONTRACTS   State Medicaid contracts with HMOs or similar managed care organizations to accept risk for a defined set of services (for example, physician services and either laboratory, x-ray, or clinic services). Other services are reimbursed on a fee-for-service basis.

PEER REVIEW Traditional quality assurance program to monitor standard processes of care or adverse outcomes of provider practice by other professional peers The goal of peer review is to find and correct medical practices that do not conform to the standard processes of care.

PER DIEM Literally, per day. Term that is applied to determining costs for a day of care and is an average that does not reflect true cost for each patient.

PER MEMBER PER MONTH (PMPM) Computational designation for each enrollee in a managed care program. It is commonly abbreviated as PMPM.

PHYSICIAN-HOSPITAL ORGANIZATION (PHO) Group practice arrangement that occurs when hospitals and physicians organize for purposes of contracting with managed care organizations. These relationships are formally organized, contractual, or corporate in character and include physicians outside the boundaries of a hospital's medical staff.

POINT-OF-SERVICE (POS) PLANS Combination of HMO and PPO features. They provide a comprehensive set of health benefits and offer a full range of health services much the same as the HMO. However, the members do not have to choose how to receive services until they need them. The member can then opt to use the defined managed care program, or can go out-of-plan for services but pay the difference for nonplan benefits (e.g., 100 percent coverage for managed care vs. 80 percent coverage out-of-plan).

PRACTICE GUIDELINES Specific, professionally agreed upon recommendation for medical practice used within or among health care organizations in an attempt to standardize practice to achieve consistent quality outcomes. Practice guidelines may be instituted when triggered by specific clinical indicators.

PREAUTHORIZATION Previous approval for specialist referral or nonemergency health care services.

PRECERTIFICATION Utilization management program that requires the individual or provider to notify the insurer before hospitalization or surgical procedure. Notification allows the insurer to authorize payment and to recommend alternate courses of action.

PREFERRED PROVIDER ORGANIZATIONS (PPOS) Managed care arrangement consisting of a group of hospitals, physicians, and other providers who have contracts with an insurer, employer, third-party administrator, or other sponsoring group to provide health care services to covered persons.

PREMIUMS Periodic payment to keep an insurance policy in force.

PREVAILING CHARGES   Amounts charged by health care providers that are consistent with charges from similar providers for identical or similar services in a given locale.

PREVENTIVE MEDICINE   Wellness and health promotion services that are part of the basic benefits package of a managed health care plan.

PRIMARY CARE   Nonspecialist, basic medical care.

PRIMARY CARE CASE MANAGEMENT   Single provider is responsible for co-ordinating, arranging, and monitoring all patient care, even for those patients with no serious medical conditions.

PRIMARY CARE PHYSICIAN (PCP)   Primary deliverers and managers of health care, central to controlling costs and utilization. The PCP provides basic care to the enrollee, initiates referrals to specialists, and provides follow-up care. Refers exclusively to other contracted providers and admits patients only to contracted hospitals. Usually defined as a physician practicing in such areas as internal medicine, family practice, and pediatrics.

PROFILING   Systematic method of collecting, collating, and analyzing patient data to develop provider-specific information about medical practice.

PROSPECTIVE REVIEW   Data-gathering technique that uses projected figures or current data to determine future costs or services.

PROTOCOL   Tool for enhancing quality in a health care organization by developing customary methods for medical interventions. Treatment protocols are developed for clinical areas of medicine where diagnostic or therapeutic approaches are well defined. Technology assessment and quality studies are used to establish decision protocols for particular diseases or treatments.

PROVIDERS   Term used to describe medical professionals and service organizations that provide health care services.

Q

QUALIFIED PROVIDER   Health care provider who has been contracted with or authorized to provide reimbursable health care services from an insurer or payor.

QUALITY ASSURANCE   Set of activities that measures the characteristics of health care services and may include corrective measures.

R

READMISSION   Patient admission to a hospital for the same or similar diagnosis as a previous, recent admission. Often used as a measure of inappropriate discharge or treatment from the first admission.

REFERRAL   Primary care physician-directed transfer of a patient to a specialty physician or specialty care.

REFERRAL POOL   Capitation set-aside for referrals or inpatient medical services. If utilization targets are met at the end of the year, primary care physicians may share what is left in the pool.

REHABILITATION   Process and goal of restoring disabled insureds to maximum physical, mental, and vocational independence and productivity commensurate with their limitations.

RESOURCE-BASED RELATIVE VALUE SCALE (RBRVS)   Developed by the Health Care Financing Administration (HCFA) of the federal government to redistribute physician payments more adequately to encourage the use of PCP services. The amount of resources devoted to produce a health care service serves as the basis for the fee that is paid.

RETROSPECTIVE CLAIM REVIEW   Examination of claim data after completion of medical services to assess appropriateness of care or reimbursement for services.

RISK   Chance of incurring financial loss by an insurer or provider.

RISK ADJUSTMENT   Correction of capitation or fee rates based upon factors that can cause an increase in medical costs such as age or sex.

RISK CONTRACT   See Medicare Risk Contract.

RISK SHARING   Apportionment of chance of incurring financial loss by insurers, managed care organizations, and health care providers.

S

SECOND SURGICAL OPINIONS   Utilization control to determine appropriateness of surgery by a second provider source.

SELF-REFERRAL   Choice by the insured or patient of medical specialists or specialty services without need for primary care physician or health plan controls.

SELF-INSURERS   Employers, businesses, and other entities that chose to assume the responsibilities of an insurance company to insure their beneficiaries.

SET-ASIDE   See Withhold Arrangements.

75/25 RULE   HMOs participating in the Medicaid program are required to limit Medicaid and Medicare recipients to no more than 75 percent of enrollees and to draw at least 25 percent of their enrollees from the private sector. This "75/25 rule" is imposed to ensure that care provided to Medicaid enrollees is comparable to that provided to enrollees with private insurance.

SKILLED NURSING FACILITIES   Institution providing the degree of medical care required from, or under the supervision of, a registered nurse or a physician.

SOCIAL SECURITY ACT   Law under which the federal government operates the Old Age, Survivors, Disability, and Health Insurance Program (OASDHI). Includes Medicare and Medicaid.

SPECIALTY MANAGED CARE ARRANGEMENTS   Those group practices and organizations of providers who contract with managed care organizations to provide nonprimary care medical services.

SPECIALTY PHYSICIANS   Those physicians practicing in areas other than internal medicine, family practice, or pediatrics.

STAFF-MODEL HMO   HMO that owns the clinical facilities used by patients enrolled in the HMO. The physicians providing service are directly employed by the HMO and they provide service only to patients enrolled in the HMO plan.

STAKEHOLDERS   Those with a stake in the cost and quality of health care services, including patients, employers, providers, and government.

STOP-LOSS INSURANCE   Protection purchased by self-insured and some managed care arrangements against the risk of large losses or severe adverse claim experience.

SUBACUTE CARE   Health care services that are less intense than hospital care but more intense than skilled nursing home services.

SUPPLEMENTARY COVERAGE   Insurance to help cover those parts of Medicare Part B that are nonreimbursable.

T

THIRD-PARTY ADMINISTRATOR   Method by which an outside person or firm, not a party to a contract, maintains all records regarding the persons covered by an insurance plan. Entity also may pay claims.

TOTAL DISABILITY   Generally, a disability that prevents insureds from performing all occupational duties.

TRIGGERS   Data point or indicator that suggests further study or review.

TRIPLE OPTION PLAN   Employer insurance plans that offer an HMO, a provider network, and a point-of-service option.

24-HOUR COVERAGE   Any combination of traditional health insurance and workers' compensation insurance that attempts to dissolve the occupational and nonoccupational boundaries between the two coverages.

U

UNBUNDLED   Health services or benefits that are a stand-alone or carved out benefit under a separate contract or bill.

UNDERWRITERS   Insurance professionals who determine if and on what basis an insurer will accept an application for insurance.

USUAL, CUSTOMARY, AND REASONABLE (UCR) FEES   Charges of health care providers that are consistent with charges from similar providers for identical or similar services in a given locale.

UTILIZATION   Patterns of usage for single medical service or type of service (hospital care, prescription drugs, physician visits). Measurement of utilization of all medical services in combination usually is done in terms of dollar expenditures. Use is expressed in rates per unit of population at risk for a given period, such as number of annual admissions to a hospital per 1,000 persons over age 65.

UTILIZATION REVIEWS (UR)   Programs designed to reduce unnecessary medical services, both inpatient and outpatient. Utilization reviews may be prospective, retrospective, concurrent, or in relation to discharge planning.

V

VENDORS   Term describing a person, persons, groups, and organizations providing health care services for reimbursement.

W

WAIVERS   Term usually associated with the Medicare or Medicaid programs by which the government waives certain regulations or rules for a managed care or insurance program to operate in a certain geographic area.

WITHHOLD ARRANGEMENTS   Portion of a provider's salary, fees, or capitation that is held back until performance in relation to quality and utilization are examined at the end of each year. If performance was at least satisfactory, withholds are released to the provider.

WORKERS' COMPENSATION   Liability insurance requiring certain employers to pay benefits and furnish medical care to employees for on-the-job injuries and to pay benefits to dependents of employees killed by occupational accidents.

WRAP-AROUND COVERAGE   Programs of HMOs that, in some states, were prevented by state law from taking on financial risk for out-of-plan care and joined with insurers to cover the out-of-plan portion of care. Such programs led to the development of point-of-service plans (POS).

INDEX

Abuse, control, 147–150
Access to care, 80–81, 102, 108
    unlimited, 33, 34, 45
Accident coverage, 110
Accreditation, 151–154
Adjusted Average per Capita Cost
        (AAPCC), 93–95
Adjusted community rate (ACR), 94
Administration, 21
    costs, 5, 111
    files, 144
    simplicity, 112
    systems, 145
Affinity analysis, 127
Agency for Health Care Policy and Re-
        search (AHCPR), 122–123
    guidelines, 122–123
Aging, 8
    military population, 104
    population, 98–99
Aid to Families with Dependent Chil-
        dren (AFDC), 103
Alternatives, selection of, 125
Ambulatory care, 35, 77, 143
American Medical Association (AMA),
        15–16, 122
Ancillary services, 77, 92
Annual benefit cap, 47
Applications reporting systems, 145
Appropriateness of care, 3–4, 10, 66,
        67–68, 70, 71, 102, 151
Appropriate use of services, 76
Attitude, American consumers, 3
Audits 148–149, 153, 154
Authorization reviews, 70, 120
Automated systems, 144–145, 148
Average length of stay, 66

Balance billing, 62, 88
Bar charts, 131
Barriers
    Medicaid population, 102
    technical and regulatory, 104
Baylor Plan, 14
Behavioral health
    data measurement, 150–151
    programs, 24–25, 44, 45
Benchmark, 124
Benchmarking, 133–134
Benefit design, 76, 113
Benefit package, 30, 82, 83
Benefits, 78, 113
    coordination, 79
    EPO, 42
    HMOs, 34
    POS, 41–43
Blue Cross/Blue Shield, 14, 22, 23
Brainstorming, 127, 130
Bulk purchasing, 46
Bundled program, 49–50
Business coalitions, 86–88

Cafeteria-type benefit plan, 49
Capital costs, 35, 36, 39
Capital markets, 20
Capitated payment arrangements, 147
Capitation, 35, 36, 41, 44, 49, 50, 56–
        57, 60–61, 93, 99, 100, 103
    PHOs, 60–61
    prepaid, 100
    rates, 88, 93, 141
Capitation risk contracts, 93
    comprehensive or full, 103
    partial, 103

Carve-outs, 44, 45, 49, 57
Case audits, 120
Case management, 41, 45, 52, 68–69, 71, 99, 106, 108
  fee, 102
  primary care physician, 16
Case rates, 61
Catastrophic cases, 37, 52, 68, 108
Causal relationship, 132
Cause-and-effect analysis, 130–131
Centers of excellence, 52
Certification, 17
  data requirements 151–154
Change, needed, 2–8
Chronic care, 44, 50, 52, 99
Civilian Health and Medical Program of the Uniformed Services (CHAMPUS), 91, 105
  demonstrations, 105
  reform initiatives, 105
Claims, 43, 47
  adjudication, 145
  data, 143, 144, 148
  screen devices, 71
Clinical indicator, 119
Clinical managers, 146
Clinical outcomes, 150
Clinical reviews, 120
Clinical systems, 145
Closed panel, 35, 36
  PCP payment, 55–58
CMM, 141
CMP Medicare programs, 94–96
Coding, 148
Coinsurance, 40, 58, 76
Collective bargaining, 15
Collective purchasing agreements, 87
Community Health Purchasing Alliance (CHPA), 113
Community-rated premiums, 84
Comparative practice patterns, 141–142
Competitive bidding, 87

Competitive medical plans (CMPs), 93
Computerized systems, 146
Concurrent review, 70, 107
  and retrospective, 88, 120
Confidentiality, 148
  codes, 148
Congress, 105–106
Congressional Budget Office, 68
Consistency, 112
Consolidated policies and benefits, 110
Consumer, 83, 118
  benefit coordination, 79
  changes, need for, 3
  choice of health plan, 77–78
  individual, 75–77
  influence on managed care, 81
  out-of-pocket expenses, 78–79
Consumer Price Index, 16, 25, 83
Continuous Quality Improvement (CQI), 118, 125–136, 153
  benefits of, 135–136
  impementation, 134–135
  methods and tools, 126–134
  QA vs, 126, 127
Contracting, 63–68
Cooperative purchasing arrangements, 77–78, 86–88
Coordinated Care Program, 105
Coordination of Benefits (COB), 79
Copayment, 20, 40, 43, 45, 47, 58, 79, 113
Correlation, 132
Cost, 83
  analysis, 146
  basis, 35, 93
  escalation, 1, 3–4, 16, 21
  per employee by plan type, 28, 29, 30
Cost containment
  mental health, 25
  workers' compensation, 108
Cost contracting, 96

Cost control, 22, 25, 105, 146
  HMO, 33, 34
  PHO, 38
  POS, 44
  PPO, 41
  techniques, 55–73
Cost-effectiveness of care, 4, 65–66,
    108, 120, 123
Cost-effectiveness of practice, 66
Cost per member per month
    ($PMPM), 141
Cost sharing, 76, 77, 78, 80, 83,
    105
Cost shifting, 2, 7
Coverage, 20
  limitations, 45
  multiple plans, 79
CQI *see* Continuous Quality Im-
    provement
Credentialing, 34, 42, 49, 64–65,
    121
Credentials, 64–65
Cumulative member month (CMM),
    141
Current procedural terminology
    (CPT), 57
Customer focus, 125
Customers, 117, 118, 136
Customer satisfaction, 81, 136, 147

Data
  deficiencies, 6–7
  sources, 143–144
  time and, 140
Database forecasting, 143
Database management systems, 145
Death benefits, 107
Decision support systems (DSS), 145
Deductibles, 20, 40, 47, 76, 77, 79,
    83, 106
  see also Out-of-pocket expenses
Defensive medicine, 2, 6

Defined provider
  networks, 97
  services, 63
Demand analysis, 146
Deming, W. Edward, 125
  chain reactions, 126
Demographic needs, need to respond,
    8
Demography, 26, 102
  see also Population trends
Demonstration projects, 101
  Department of Defense, 105
  requirements, 104
Denial of payment, 120
Dental specialty programs, 46–49
  coverage, 47
Department of Defense health pro-
    grams, 91
Designated
  providers, 108
  PCP, 58
DHMO *see* Health Maintenance Organi-
    zations, dental
Diagnosis-related group (DRG), 61–
    62
Disability benefits, 107, 109, 110,
    111
Disability management, 112
Disability, partial, 107
Disability, total, 107
Discharge planning, 71, 88
Discount, 57
Discounted fee-for-service basis, 36,
    41, 42, 47, 50
Discounted fee schedules, 88
Discounted per diem, 88
Discounted RBRVS rates, 59, 63
Disease coverage, 110
Disenrollment, right to, 103
Double-dipping, 112
Drug utilization review, 46
Duplicate payments, avoidance,
    112

Education cost-effective use of health care system, 87, 102

Effectiveness, measures of, 29–30

Elderly, the, 95, 99
see also Population trends

Emergency room services, 76–77

Employee Assistance Program (EAP), 45

Employee choices, 82–84, 113

Employers
large, 85
managed care and, 81–86
small, 85–86, 112–113

Enrollees, 9, 81
Medicaid and HMOs, 100, 101
Medicaid and Medicare, 101

Enrollment, 18, 21, 22, 23, 94, 95
CHAMPUS, 105
FEHBP, 105
HIPC, 112–113
Medicaid, 104
regional variation, 25–27
rural United States, 28–29

Environmental factors, 52–53

Evaluation, 125

Excess capacity, 2

Exclusive Provider Organization (EPO), 22, 42, 67, 86

Expectations, 67

Expected benefits, 24-hour services, 111–112

Expenses, HMO, 21

Experience-rated groups, 98

Experience-rated premiums, 84

Federal Employee Health Benefits Program (FEHBP), 105–106
reforms, 106

Federally qualified, 17

Feedback process, 139, 143

Fee-for-service, 3–5, 34, 36, 42, 43, 47, 57–60, 78, 84, 100, 103
discounts, 20
Medicare, 93, 94
medicine, 13, 16, 30
PCP, 56
PHO, 59–60
plans, 106

Fees
schedules, 62–63
usual, customary, and reasonable, 47

Financial performance, 142

Financial risk, 33, 35, 36, 39, 44, 49, 93
DRG, 61–62
PHO, 59

Fishbone diagram, 130

Fixed payment, 102–103

Fixed percentage, premium cost, 83

Fixed premium, 34

Flow charts, 128–129

Focus groups, 136

FOCUS-PDCA, 134–135

Forerunners, 14–15

Formulary, 46, 149

Fraud, 7
control, 147–150

Freedom-of-choice, 100, 101, 103

Freestanding plan, 49

Frequency, 146, 153

Gantt charts, 132

Garfield, Sidney, 15

Gatekeeper, 16, 34, 41, 43, 67

General Accounting Office (GAO), 25, 96

General Motors, 17

Generic drugs, 46

Global fees, 57–58
Government
  changes, need for, 6–8
  involvement, 91–116
Grand Coulee Dam workers, 15
Gross Margin PMPM, 142
Group Health Association of America (GHAA), 95
Group Health of Minneapolis, 20
Group medical catastrophe coverage, 15
Group medical coverages, 110–111
Group-model HMO, 15, 18, 35
Group practices, 35
  without walls, 38
Group-only, 97–98
Guidelines, 45
  clinical practice, 122–123
  Medicaid, 101

Health benefits, 17
  World War II, 15–16
Health care delivery system, 4
Health Care Financing Administration (HCFA), 59, 94, 97, 144
  Medicaid requirements, 101
  Medicare reimbursement, 94, 95
Health Care Quality Improvement Act of 1986, 66
Health care prepayment plans (HCPP), 97
Health Insurance Plan of California (HIPC), 112–113
Health-insuring organizations, 103
Health Maintenance Organization (HMO), 14, 34–52, 67, 78, 106, 107
  dental, 49–50
  development loans and grants, 17
  employer influence, 84
  federally qualified, 100
  Group-model, 15, 18, 22, 35–36
  group-only, 97–98
  managed care alliance, 113
  Medicare and, 94–96
  membership, 98
  Mixed-model, 39–40
  models, 35–40
  national firms, 22
  open-ended, 20
  operation of, 34
  preventive care, 80
  risk contracts, 93–95
  state government employees, 106–107
Health Maintenance Organization (HMO) Act of 1973, 17–19, 82, 91, 93, 105
Health Plan Employer Data and Information Set (HEDIS) 2.0, 154
Health policy, employers and, 84
Health resources
  conserving, 83
  supply, 7–8
Health status, 80
Holistic approach, 108
Home health services, 45, 50
Hospice, 50, 52
Hospital days per 1,000 enrollees, 142
Hospital expense PMPM, 142
Hospitalization, 14
  alternatives, 50
  nonemergency, 77
Hospital privileges, 119–120
Hospitals, 24
  admissions, 70
  bill audit, 88
  insurance, 13, 14
  length of stay, 45, 70
  PPS, 4
  readmission rates, 144
  selection, 64, 65

services, 92, 93
utilization, 108, 142
utilization management, 69

Impact areas, 128
Implementation, 125
Incentives, 3–4
payments, 42, 43, 47
Incurred but not reported claims
(IBNR), 142
Indemnity
controls for hospital care, 77
plans, 106–107
Indemnity insurance *see* Traditional indemnity insurance
Indicator measurement system
(IMSystsem), 153
Indicators, 153
Individual Practice Association (IPA),
15, 18–19, 36–37, 94
HMOs, 58
Initial assessment, 124
Inpatient care alternatives, 16
Input, 127, 128
INPUTS-PROCESS-OUTPUTS, 139
Insolvency, 93
Insurance industry, 23
managed care and, 21–22, 23
Insureds' wages, 83
Insurer, 44
response to managed care, 21–23
Integrated coverage, 109–110
Integrated delivery system, 38
Integrated multiple options, 23
Integrated policies and benefits, 109,
110
Integrated services, 109
IPA *see* Individual Practice Association

Joint Commission on Accreditation of
Healthcare Organizations
(JCAHO), 151, 152–153

Kaiser, Henry J., 15
Kaiser Permanente Medical Care Program, 15
Kaoru Ishikawa, 130

Laboratory reports, 144
Labor unions, 15, 86
Legislation, 15, 20
24-hour pilots, 112
Legislative barriers, 6
Liability
insurance, 49
limit calculation, 37
Licensure
HMOs, 17
see also Credentialing
Lifestyle, 80
Limited-service models, 44
Litigation, 6, 118, 147
Long-term care, 98–99
Loos, H. Clifford, 14
Loss of earnings benefits, 107

Malpractice, 2, 4, 6, 66, 120, 121
Managed care, 8–9
alliances, 112–113
culture, 26–27
current marketplace, 23–30
defined, 9
demonstration projects, 99
employer influence, 81–86
enrollee satisfaction, 81
factors affecting, 52–53
factors affecting need for, 1–2
features, 9, 33–34
growth of, 18–20, 21
information types, 141–142
investment in, 22–23
long-term care and, 98–99
organization of, 33–54
traditional insurance vs, 9–10

Managed indemnity, 52
Managed mental health, 20, 24–25
Managed pharmacy programs, 20, 25
Managed Risk Medical Insurance
    Board (MRMIB), 113
Management Information Systems
    (MIS), 145–147
  fraud and abuse, 147–149
  other, 147
Management Services Organization
    (MSO), 38
Mandated benefits, 6
Marketing program, 109
Mayo Clinic, 13, 14
Medicaid, 2, 7, 91, 99–104
  benefits, 99
  eligibility, 99, 103–104
  enrollment, 100
  history, 100
  population, expanding managed
    care, 104
  requirements waived, 101
  restrictions, 100
Medical and disability coverage, 110
Medical benefits, 107
Medical board examinations, 121
Medical coverage 109, 110
Medical foundation, 38
Medical management, 21, 23, 112
Medical necessity, 68
Medical practice patterns, 3–4, 9
Medical record review, 66
Medical records, 148
Medical service bureau, 13
Medical societies, 15–16
Medicare, 2, 7, 91, 92–95
  HMOs, 94–96
  managed care and, 99
  Part A, 92, 93
  Part B, 92, 93, 96, 97
  POS, 97
  PPS, 4
  qualified providers, 93

Medicare SELECT, 96–97
  demonstrations, 97
MedSup, 96–97
Membership see Enrollment
Mental health case management pro-
    gram, 101
Mental health management, 40, 45
Mental health services, 85
Military Health Services System
    (MHSS), 104–105
Montgomery Ward and Company, his-
    tory, 13
Multiple provider arrangement, 39
Multispecialty clinics, 58
Multispecialty group practice, 13, 35,
    52
Mutual benefit society, 14

National Association of Insurance
    Commissioners (NAIC), 17, 109
National Committee on Quality Assur-
    ance (NCQA), 151, 153–154
National Labor Relations Board
    (NLRB), 15
National Practitioner Data Bank, 66
Negotiated fees, 40, 41, 42, 47, 57,
    60, 61
Netherlands, coverage, 110
Network, 34, 38, 42, 45, 46, 47, 49,
    63, 87, 149, 153
  HMO, 39–40, 43, 49
  utilization, 112
Network providers, 20, 78, 85
New Jersey Commission on Income
    Maintenance in 1980, 109
New Zealand Accident Compensation
    system, 110
Nonemergency inpatient care, 106
Non-network provider see Out-of-plan
    care
Nonprofit foundation, 38
Norms of practice, 70

Occupational injuries, 107, 108
Office of Personnel Management (OPM), 105
Omnibus Budget Reconciliation Act (OBRA), 96, 100, 101, 106
Open-ended HMO, 20
Open panel, 36
Organizational risk, 121
Other expenses PMPM, 142
Outcome management, 119
Outcome measurement, 66, 119
Outcome measures, data for, 151
Outcomes, 125, 128
Out-of-plan care, 20, 21, 22, 40, 41, 42-43, 44, 58, 78
Out-of-pocket expenses, 58, 75, 76, 77, 78-79, 82, 83
  see also Deductibles
Outpatient care, 45
Outpatient forecasting, 142
Outpatient precertification, 70
Outputs, 139
Overutilization, 62, 76-77, 93, 120, 147
  see also Utilization. . .

Pareto chart, 133
Partial hospitalization, 45
Passwords, 148
Patient records, 148
Patient satisfaction surveys, 121, 150
Payers, 118
  need for changes, 4-5
Payment for services, HMOs, 34-35
Payment levels, Medicare, 98
PDCA continuous model, 136
Peer review, 120, 121
  committee, 34
Per diem, 61
Performance, 58, 63
  criteria, 45
Performance reports, 150

Per member per month (PMPM), 56-57, 61, 141
Per member per year (PMPY), 141
Pharmaceutical services, 46
Pharmacy networks, 46
Physician associations, 15
Physician expense PMPM, 142
Physician-Hospital Organization (PHO), 37-39, 59-63
  ownership, 37
Physician peer review, 16
Physician profile, 63, 65-66
Physicians, 24
  education, 4
  IPA-model HMOs, 18-19
  number of, 17-18
  reimbursement, 3-4
  role in medical resource usage, 3-4
Physician services, 92, 93
Physician specialties, 108
Pie charts, 131-132
Plan design, 78-79
Planning, 124
Point-of-Service (POS) Plan, 20-21, 26, 42-44, 49, 78-79, 84, 86, 97
Population trends, 8, 98-99
  military, 104
Practice guideline, 119, 122-123
Practice parameters, 122
Practice patterns, 9, 35, 36, 39, 49, 120, 121
Practice profile see Physician profile
Practice standard, 119, 123
Preadmission certification, 52, 69-70 106
Preadmission review, 88, 120
Preapproval, 58
Pre-approval, nonemergency hospitalization, 16, 58, 108
Preauthorization, 70, 108
Precertification, 23, 88, 106, 108, 120
Preferred benefits, 113

Preferred Provider Organization (PPO), 14–15, 20, 22 , 23–24, 40–41, 67, 78–79, 85–86, 97, 106, 108–109
  dental, 47
  employer influence, 84
  IPA-model vs, 20, 21–22
  managed care alliance, 113
  Medicare, 97
  plans, 79, 86
  reimbursement, 41
  simple discount, 58
  state government employees, 106–107
Premiums, 10, 34–35, 45, 81
  HIPC, 113
  HMO rates, 21
  state-paid, 103
  workers' compensation, 107
Premium sharing
  employer-employee, 82–84
  fixed percentage, 83
  traditional, 81
Prepaid group practices, 14, 15, 16
Prepayment, 10, 14, 15, 16
  dental plans, 49
Prescription drugs, 25
Prescription drugs specialty programs, 44, 46
Prevailing charges, 7
Preventive
  medicine, 5
  services, 57
Preventive care, 43, 57, 79–81
  consumers and, 3
Primary care, 58
Primary care case management, 100, 102
Primary care physician (PCP), 34, 36, 39, 40, 41, 43, 55–56, 67, 77, 78, 79
  payment, closed panels, 55–58
Priorities, 123–124

Private practice, 36, 39
Problem identification, 124
Problem solving, 123–125
Process change, 135
Processes, 128, 139
Productivity improvement, 137
Productivity reports, 146
Professional review, 45, 49
Profiling, 142, 143–144
Profit margin, 142
Prospective capitation, 93
Prospective data analysis, 148
Prospective screening, 16
Prospective utilization review, 69–70, 77
Protocols, 45
  decision, 70
Provider networks, 84, 97
Providers, 3–4, 20
  need for changes, 3–4
  selection, 63–67
Public assistance, 99–104
Public Law 89-97, 7

Qualifications, HMO and Medicaid, 100
Quality, 117, 118, 122
  controlling, 117–138
  requirements, 103
Quality assurance (QA), 41, 43, 117, 118, 119–121, 146
  committees, 146
  CQI and, 126, 127
  studies, 123–125
Quality improvement (QI), 117, 118, 125, 137
  teams, 146
Quality review, 103

Rates, 135, 141–142
Rate-setting mechanisms, 104
Rate variation, 113
Ratios, 142

Readmission, 71
Reasonable cost basis, 97
Recredentialling process, 121
Red flags, 148, 149, 150
Referrals, 43, 58, 79
   authorizations, 58, 70
   patterns, 121
   pool, 57
   see also Self-referrals
Regional medical organizations, 153
Regulations, 17
Regulators, 118
Regulatory barriers, 6
Rehabilitation facilities, 50
Reimbursement system, 4–5, 55–59
   physicians, 4
Report card system, 153, 154
Resource-Based Relative Value Scale
   (RBRVS), 59
   discounted rates, 59, 63
Retrospective data analysis, 148
Retrospective reviews, 71, 120, 124,
   136
Retrospective utilization review, 71
Return to work, earlier, 112
Risk arrangements, 60–61
Risk contractors, 95
Risk contracts, 93, 102–103
   full capitation, 103
   HMO, 93–95
   Medicare, 93, 98
   partial capitation, 103
   prepaid, 93
   TEFRA, 94
Risk factors, 143
   adjusted, 94, 151
Risk, financial, 20
Risk sharing, 36, 41, 43
Ross, Donald E., 14
Ross-Loos Clinic, 14

Salary, PCP, 56
Scatter diagrams, 132

Secondary payer, 79
Second surgical opinions, 16, 106
SELECT *see* Medicare. . .
Selection control, 63–66
Selective case management, 150–151
Selective provider relationship, 14–
   15
Self-insurers, 107
Self-referral, 41, 58, 67
Sentinel events, 153
Sentinel review, 120
75/25 rule, 101, 102, 103, 104
Sherman Antitrust Act, 16
Simplification, 112
Simple discount PPOs, 58
Single-service HMOs and PPOs, 44–50
Single-visit authorizations, 70
Site review, 121
Skilled nursing facilities, 50
Social Health Maintenance Organiza-
   tions (SHMOs), 99
Social Security Act, 92
Solo practitioners, 15
Southern California Edison, 14
Specialists, PPS, 4
Specialty care, 34, 36, 40, 41, 50–51,
   58, 63
   HMOs, 44
   managed care arrangements, 25
   reimbursement, 51
   reimbursement, 58–59
Speciality services, 58
Staff model HMO, 15, 33, 36, 49
Stakeholders, 53, 55, 56, 118
"Stand-alone" choice, 78
Standard practice, 4
Standards of care, 124
States
   government employee health bene-
     fits programs, 106–107
   insurance programs, 106–113
   medical examination board, 64, 66
   Medicaid programs, 102

monitoring, 103
welfare, 103
Stop-loss, 37
Subacute care, 50
Substance abuse services, 45, 88
  Medicaid, 101
Supplemental health insurance for
  Medicare beneficiaries (MedSup),
  96–97
Supplementary coverage, 49
Systems modeling, 127–128, 139

Tax Equity and Fiscal Responsibility
  Act (TEFRA) of 1982, 93, 94–96
Tax law, 15
Technological advances, new ap-
  proaches, 5
Technology assessment, 122
Therapeutic equivalent, 46
Third-party administrator, 40, 42
Third-party vendors, 20, 23, 45
Total IBNR per members 142
Total quality management (TQM),
  118, 125–135
Traditional indemnity insurance, 5, 9–
  10, 13, 22, 23, 33, 42, 44–45, 47,
  76, 77, 78, 79, 81–82, 93, 113
  cost, 82
  managed care vs, 9–10
Treatment protocols, 122–123
Tree diagram, 130–131
Triggers, 150, 153
Triple option plan, 106
Twenty-four-hour coverage, 109–112
  accidents, 110
  disability, 109, 110
  diseases, 110
  expected benefits, 111–112
  marketing program, 109
  medical, 109, 110
  medical and disability, 110
Twenty-four-hour services, 110

Unbundled programs, 49–50
Underutilization, 62, 150
Underwriters, 23, 103
Uniform premium rate, 94
Usual, customary, and reasonable fees,
  47
Utilization, 6, 23, 67, 95
  controls, 21, 77, 105, 146
  patterns, 120, 121
  rates, 141
Utilization management, 33, 34, 36,
  38, 39, 40, 43, 45, 52, 69, 82, 87,
  88, 97
Utilization review (UR), 6, 9, 20,
  40, 41, 43, 45, 47, 52, 67–71,
  84, 120
  inpatient, 69
  organization, 68
  postpayment, 71

Variation, 143
Volume purchasing, 87
Voluntary certification process,
  17

Waivers, Medicaid, 101
Welfare reform, 104
Wellness programs, 79–81
Withhold arrangements, 36, 37, 41,
  42, 56, 60, 120
Workers' Compensation, 91
Workers' compensation programs,
  107–112
  benefits and costs, 107
Workplace injuries see Occupational
  injuries
World War II, health benefits and,
  15–16
Wrap-around coverage, 20

Xerox Corporation, 85